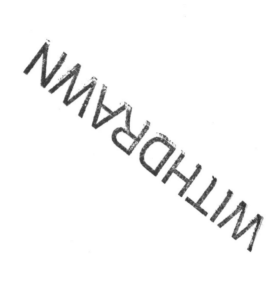

Cheating Death

The Doctors and Medical Miracles that Are
Saving Lives Against All Odds

SANJAY GUPTA, MD

with research by Caleb Hellerman

**WELLNESS
CENTRAL**

NEW YORK   BOSTON

Wellness Central
Hachette Book Group
237 Park Avenue
New York, NY 10017

Visit our website at www.HachetteBookGroup.com.

Wellness Central is an imprint of Grand Central Publishing.

The Wellness Central name and logo are trademarks
of Hachette Book Group, Inc.

Printed in the United States of America

First Edition: October 2009

10 9 8 7 6 5 4 3 2 1

Library of Congress Cataloging-in-Publication Data

Gupta, Sanjay.
Cheating death / Sanjay Gupta with research by Caleb Hellerman.
p. cm.
ISBN 978-0-446-50887-2 (regular edition)—
ISBN 978-0-446-55800-6 (large print edition)
1. Resuscitation.   2. Death, Apparent.   I. Title.
RC87.9.G87 2009
616.02'5—dc22
2009018588

For those living at the edge of a new frontier, working tirelessly to push forward the line between life and death. And for Sage, Sky and Soleil, the reasons I cheat death every day. They know it is not about eternal life, but about an extraordinary life.

Contents

Cheating
Death

Prologue

I don't want to achieve immortality through my work.
I want to achieve it through not dying.

—Woody Allen

I'M GOING TO let you in on a little secret: When the heart stops beating, it's not the end. In fact, you might say that your troubles have only just begun. As it turns out, life and death is not a black-and-white issue. There is a gray zone—a faint no-man's-land where you are neither truly dead nor actually alive. In order to control it, in order to cheat death, we have to first better understand it.

THE LAST THING Zeyad Barazanji remembers is the silence.[1] Thirty seconds earlier, he had been watching election returns on CNN, his head turned up from the treadmill, where he was huffing and puffing through his daily afternoon workout. His attention had drifted from the television to the sound of his own pounding feet, the whir of the machine, and his rasping breath as he strained to match his usual pace. That Tuesday, it felt like he was running uphill, and Barazanji cut it short, turning off the machine after only twenty minutes of jogging. A retired literature professor, Barazanji was in a bustling gym near his home in the Spuyten Duyvil section of the Bronx, surrounded by the banter of his neighbors and the clanking of weights. But then, nothing. Silence.

He doesn't remember what happened next, only what people told him later. One woman will never forget it. One minute she was working out, and the next there was a blur in the corner of her eye. The wiry, older man with the white undershirt and headband crumpled in a heap at the foot of the adjacent treadmill. At least a dozen people saw him go down. Two called 911 from their cell phones. An athletic trainer, the gym's manager, Juan Echevarria, grabbed the automatic defibrillator off the wall and rushed to Barazanji's side.

Elbowing the crowd aside, Echevarria kneeled and placed the defibrillator's electrodes on Barazanji's chest. Upon getting a signal from the device, he sent a shock into the chest of the unconscious man. Two successive bursts of electricity—200 joules apiece—shook the crumpled body. Each jolt ran through the beaded sweat on Barazanji's chest, through the breastbone, and into his still heart, shocking the muscle into a contraction. Another contraction followed, and then another. As the trainer held his breath, Barazanji's heart caught a beat of its own. The heartbeat was back. The line between life and death had shifted just enough.

The professor groaned and remained senseless, but his heart was once again sending weak pulses of blood through his sixty-three-year-old arteries. About four minutes later, a team of emergency medical technicians raced across the basketball court, stretcher in hand, to Barazanji's side. Two minutes later, a breathing tube was down his throat, he was on the stretcher, and the paramedics were sweeping toward the exit.

WE'RE USED TO thinking about dying in stark terms: dead or alive. You're here and then you're gone. In our imagination, this is how the moment of death plays out: The villain or hero or soldier gasping last words, stretching out a hand...until his eyes roll back in his head and we know it's all over. Or the cancer patient surrounded by family. A light flickers behind her eyes and then goes out. You've read it in a thousand stories, seen it in a thousand movies, a hundred episodes of *ER*. The alarm sounds. The monitor flatlines. Time of death, 2:15 a.m.

It only takes a few minutes for life to slip away. Without a heartbeat, circulation slows to a halt. Blood no longer flows to your brain or any other organ. It takes just a couple of minutes before everything goes dim, and you're blissfully unaware of the catastrophe unfolding inside your body. Starved of blood, the first organ to suffer is the brain, which in happier times consumes about 20 percent of all oxygen the body takes in, though it constitutes just 2 percent of our body mass. After ten seconds without oxygen, the brain's function slows. Without oxygen or signals from the brain, other organs break down as well. Diaphragm muscles no longer contract and release to bring in air. The kidneys stop filtering blood. At the same time, an elaborate chain of chemical reactions triggers a breakdown in cells throughout the body.

This is the process of dying. Whether because of a car accident, a blockage in an artery, or a tumor somewhere in your body, it is generally understood that when the heart stops beating, life has ended. I have seen this play out more times than I care to remember. The first time, I was a third-year medical student at the University of Michigan. The patient was not much older than I was. I remember the call coming over the emergency radio: "Twenty-three-year-old unrestrained driver in an MVA [motor vehicle accident], found with the windshield starred and steering wheel bent." Even then, I knew those details were important; it takes a lot of force to bend a steering wheel with your chest or smash a windshield with your head. I remember the trauma surgeons, neurosurgeons and orthopedic surgeons descending on this young man. They attempted to replace blood, stop bleeding and relieve pressure in his brain. It was a whirlwind of activity until . . . his heart stopped. And then everything else stopped, too. Everyone knew that was the end. After all, that's what we were taught in medical school and throughout our training. But what if it doesn't have to be that way? What if there were a way to give that twenty-three-year-old man and millions like him just a little more time, to shift the line between life and death? Ever since I watched that young man die, I have pondered that very question: can we move the line?

SURROUNDED BY FRIENDS and family in his Bronx apartment, Zeyad Barazanji told me his story of cheating death in a warm, friendly way. Barazanji, a translator and retired

Columbia professor, immigrated here from Syria back in the 1970s. His two-bedroom apartment was filled with artwork and mementos from a lifetime of traveling between New York and the Middle East. A delicious smell was in the air; his wife Raoua was whipping up a feast of Syrian delicacies and dinner was almost ready. I leaned in to listen over the buzz of activity and clinking glasses in the kitchen. We were interrupted more than once as Barazanji got up to answer the door, clapping friends on the back and hanging their coats.

It was hard to believe that this man, so full of life, was dead not long ago, but that's exactly what happened. His heart pumped no blood, his brain sent no signals, he thought no thoughts. Make no mistake—this is death. But maybe not the way we tend to think about it.

For all that's been said about immediate death—"I'm sorry, she was killed instantly"—in truth, there's no such thing. As a doctor, I can assure you that when the heart stops beating, it's not the end. Death is not a single event, but a process that may be interrupted, even reversed. And here's the exciting part—at any point during this process, the course of what seems inevitable *can* be changed. That is precisely what we are going to explore in this book: the possibility of cheating death.

As the ambulance screeched away from the curb in front of Bally's Total Fitness, Barazanji was in the gray zone—not dead but not quite fully alive, either. Millions of cells in his heart were already dead, suffocated by a lack of blood flow. It was too soon to say whether the damage was enough to cause a broader failure, similar to the collapse of a wall from which termites have taken one too many nibbles. It was also too soon to say if a significant number of brain cells—cells which had been nourished by a constant diet of oxygen for more than sixty-three years—had starved in those first precious minutes. There was no way to know just yet if the march toward death might be reversed.

Barazanji could easily be you or me, our father or mother. In a sense, what happened to Barazanji is extraordinary, but in another sense, it happens to us all eventually. It's been said that life is a terminal condition, that nothing lasts forever, and the minute we're born, we start the long process of our end. I think everyone, at one point or another, has probably wondered: does it really have to be that way? When we explore the story of Barazanji, we're exploring the chances of cheating death—for you or me.

What you're holding in your hands is a medical thriller that explores an exciting and fast-moving realm of science. In these pages, we'll take you to the thin line that separates life and death, along with the doctors who struggle to keep their patients on the right side of the line. We will also explore that border through the eyes and ears of people who have found themselves straddling it, and we'll introduce you to scientists who are taking on incredible challenges. These determined pioneers are true optimists who believe that even if we don't yet have all the answers, we may find them.

From womb to deathbed, we'll see the myriad ways that modern science is changing our understanding of life and death. You'll see that neither the starting nor the finish line is written in stone; they are written in sand, shifting with each new wave of medical understanding and technology. In our journey to understand death—and to find a way to stave it off—we're going to explore the gray no-man's-land between this life and whatever lies beyond it.

Before we tell what happened to Barazanji, we're going to introduce you to another explorer, a woman who has been to the no-man's-land and lived to tell the tale. She arrived there by accident, on a faraway mountainside, in a world where people are used to working and playing in bitter cold and near darkness. That mountainside is the first stop on our remarkable journey.

CHAPTER ONE

Ice Doctors

She presented all the ordinary appearances of death.
The face assumed the usual pinched and sunken
outline. The lips were of the usual marble pallor. The
eyes were lusterless. There was no warmth. Pulsation
had ceased.

—Edgar Allan Poe, "The Premature Burial"

IN MAY 1999, a twenty-nine-year-old medical resident, Anna Bagenholm, was skiing with two friends near Narvik in northern Norway. They were colleagues as well as friends. All three were training at nearby Narvik Hospital, a small community hospital. Torvind Næsheim was working toward becoming an anesthesiologist, who handles the duties of an emergency physician in Norway. Marie Falkenberg hoped to be a pediatric surgeon.[1]

Bagenholm was studying to become an orthopedic surgeon. An experienced backcountry skier, she had chosen to work in Narvik in part because of the spectacular mountains where she could ski nearly year-round. That fateful day, she and her friends had hiked about 30 minutes into an off-piste area, a place they had come many times before. They soon were making their way down a gully carved by a stream, now frozen and coated with a thin layer of snow. Largely hidden from the sun, the spot was known as the Mørkhåla, or black hole.

The details of the accident were wiped from Bagenholm's memory by the months that followed, but somehow she fell and found herself sliding on her back. To her friends, it looked at first like a run-of-the mill tumble, but when they came closer, they could see that Bagenholm had broken partly through some ice and was trapped.

She was wedged headfirst between rocks and an overhanging shelf of ice that capped the stream rushing over her head. From what Falkenberg and Næsheim could tell, Bagenholm was in an air pocket, because she was still moving. There was no time to lose. They tried to tug her free, each hanging on to a leg, but the current pulled back and the cold made it difficult to keep a firm grip. After seven minutes they gave up and used a cell phone to call for help. The dispatcher at Narvik, a colleague, told them help was on the way, but it was a difficult wait, watching as Bagenholm's struggles grew weaker and then ceased. It had been forty minutes since her head plunged through the ice.

By then, fellow skiers and friends were on the scene. Nearly forty minutes after that, at 7:39 p.m., another friend arrived with a steel garden shovel. Along with Næsheim and Falkenberg, they cut a hole through thick ice a short ways downstream, attached a rope to Bagenholm's leg and dragged her underwater to the new hole, where they pulled her from the water.

Photos taken at the scene show a lifeless body, the pallor of its blue skin broken only by some dull purple welts and the pale oxygen lines. Bagenholm was soaking wet and by traditional measures, clinically dead. Næsheim and Falkenberg were experienced in backcountry medicine and weren't ready to give up. They immediately commenced CPR. A few minutes later, a second medical team arrived by helicopter. The chopper hovered above while a rescuer dropped down, secured Bagenholm's airway and strapped her to a backboard so she could be winched up to the helicopter. By 7:56 p.m., she was en route to the University of North Norway Hospital in Tromso, about 150 miles away.

As they soared through the darkening sky, the rescuers took turns pumping Bagenholm's chest, using the desperate rhythm of CPR. The young physician still showed no sign of life. She had no breath, no pulse. A thermometer revealed that her core body temperature was just 56 degrees Fahrenheit.

Stick your foot in a bucket of 56-degree water, and in less than a minute, it will start to hurt. If you jump into water that is 56 degrees Fahrenheit, it will suck the breath out of you. Stay in the water for ten minutes, and you'll be suffering from hypothermia. Bagenholm had been in the water for more than an hour, and she was in the air, in the rescue chopper, for another hour and fourteen minutes.

There was only one real glimmer of hope. There's a

saying in medicine that no one is dead until they are warm and dead. Bagenholm would not be warm for a long, long time. The rescue team knew that the very cold that was killing this young woman could end up saving her, too. They knew they had science on their side, as long as they could be patient. Instead of throwing blankets on Bagenholm and infusing warm IV fluid, they sat back, and waited.

The idea that cold might improve the chance of survival was truly discovered by accident, but it's a lesson that's driven home on a regular basis. Some recent examples: In the spring of 2008, a forty-three-year-old British woman named Mandy Evans survived after falling off a mountainous footpath and ending up in a near-freezing river; she lay there nine hours before rescuers found her. Her body temperature had fallen to 77 degrees Fahrenheit. In 2001, a Canadian toddler survived a night when her body temperature dropped to less than 58 degrees Fahrenheit. She had slipped out the front door of her home on a midwinter night, and then couldn't get the door back open. She was found the next morning and rushed to the hospital; she eventually made a full recovery.[2]

As these examples make obvious, under certain conditions the body can dramatically modify its requirements for survival. Doctors have long explored ways to make use of this lifesaving principle. Therapeutic hypothermia was first used in the 1940s and 1950s, when pioneering heart surgeons like Walt Lillehei started using hypothermia to extend their time in the operating room. Prior to the 1940s, most open-heart surgeries were thought to be impossible, because anything more than a very simple repair could not be completed in the few minutes that the heart—and brain—might survive without oxygen. By chilling a patient's blood, Lillehei found that he could buy precious minutes. A heart that only lasted ten minutes at room temperature could survive an hour when it was cooled to 20 degrees Celsius.[3]

There's no easy answer as to how or why hypothermia really works. The first person I thought to ask was Dr. Lance Becker, an emergency physician and researcher who runs the Center for Resuscitation Science at the University of Pennsylvania School of Medicine. Becker says the hypothermia procedure is still mysterious. "We're pretty sure it doesn't work on just one mechanism. I've looked at twenty or thirty ideas [in the lab] that have been postulated, but the truth is, nobody knows [just why or how it helps]."

What does seem clear is that as a medical therapy, hypothermia buys time. I explain it this way: Chest compressions and artificial respiration provide oxygen that the body needs, but hypothermia slows the body down. That in turn reduces the need for oxygen, so the body can last longer on what's already there.

Studies show that every 1 degree (Celsius) drop in body temperature will lower cellular metabolism by roughly 5 to 7 percent.[4] Becker's best guess is that this reduced metabolism also slows the chemical reactions that are triggered by oxygen deprivation and which prove so damaging to cells. There's no doubt this is complicated. Hibernation is a good example of cold going hand in hand with lower metabolism; mammals who hibernate can survive, even thrive, for long periods of time at far below their usual body temperature. In these animals, cold doesn't just slow metabolism the way it thickens a jar of molasses. Rather, it triggers a whole set of biochemical changes.

Hibernation seems to be caused by different factors, depending on the animal, but cold weather is a common trigger. Take ground squirrels, for example. As soon as temperatures dip below freezing on a regular basis, ground squirrels go into a near-complete torpor. Their heart rate, usually around two hundred beats per minute, slows to less than ten. The squirrel's body temperature will drop from a warm-blooded 37 degrees Celsius to just one or two degrees above the outside temperature. They stay in that state, using just a bare minimum of energy, for at least six months.[5]

True, humans aren't squirrels, but believe it or not, we have some of the same adaptive ability. For example, immersion in cold water triggers something called the mammalian diving reflex. You could think of it as throwing the body into a state of semi-hibernation. Blood flow is shunted from the extremities to the heart and lungs, breathing slows, and the heart and brain use less than half of the oxygen they normally require. Survival time is stretched out.

BAGENHOLM COULDN'T HAVE known it at the time, but as the helicopter prepared to land, her life was about to intersect with a doctor who in one way or another had been preparing for this moment all his professional life. The director of emergency services at the University Hospital in Tromso was Dr. Mads Gilbert. Like his patient, Gilbert is a daredevil, a risk taker, enjoying off-piste skiing and trekking through the wilderness. He loves action; he loves riding the emergency helicopters that serve as ambulances for much of the far-flung, mountainous stretch of coastal Norway that surrounds his home base. In fact he had taken off in the rescue chopper to treat Bagenholm in the field, and only turned back when he learned that a larger, better-equipped helicopter was closer to the scene.

Gilbert spends his vacation time in places like Burma and Kurdistan, teaching emergency medical techniques to people who don't live anywhere near a hospital and doctors who have to treat battlefield wounds with only the barest medical kits. He had a brush with worldwide fame in 2008, during Israel's offensive in the Gaza Strip. Gilbert was interviewed inside a Gaza hospital, where he helped to treat wounded fighters and civilians. He accused Israel of deliberately killing civilians and in turn was denounced by conservative critics who called him a "Hamas apologist" and a "shill for terrorism."[6]

In other words, Gilbert is not a man who shies from controversy, whether the debate is over politics or medicine. That was true long before he started turning up in global hot spots. Some might consider his risk taking dangerous, even reckless, but in Bagenholm's case, it was exactly what she needed. Many other doctors would have given up, and for good reason. Taking stock of his new patient, Gilbert told me he knew that she didn't look good. "I saw this very,

very athletic young girl. But she looked like a corpse." By the time Anna Bagenholm was wheeled into the operating room, she had been clinically dead for three hours.

When I first read about the Bagenholm case, I imagined a daring physician, attempting extravagant new measures on behalf of his beautiful, hopeless patient. I imagined only sheer desperation would drive someone to that brink of attempting the impossible. As it turns out, only some of this is true. The effort to save Bagenholm did in fact stem from desperation, but it was not so much a matter of luck as careful guesswork and experience.

Before the Bagenholm rescue, Gilbert says his team had made at least fifteen previous attempts to resuscitate patients with no pulse and severe accidental hypothermia.[7] They were fishermen or skiers or hikers who had fallen in the sea or through ice, or gotten trapped under snow, or simply become drunk and lost in the woods until they nearly froze to death. When I asked Gilbert how many of those patients had survived, he looked away for a second and then replied thoughtfully, "We hadn't succeeded with a single survivor, but we were getting closer and closer." He told me, "In fact, the person just before Anna was in some ways an even more dramatic story."

Just a few months earlier, Gilbert had flown a risky helicopter mission to the scene of an avalanche that had buried another skier, a young university student. The student and a companion had set off the avalanche while telemarking down a pristine snowfield near the base of Ullstinden, a popular ski mountain just north of Tromso. The student's companion managed to avoid the collapse and made it down to the road to seek help. In the meantime, two young skiers who had seen the accident from above made it down to the scene and began to dig.

Gilbert's rescue chopper arrived within the hour, but the side of the valley was too steep for it to land, so the helicopter touched down on a ridge several hundred yards above. Gilbert, a nurse, and a local police officer clambered down the side of the valley. By the time they reached the victim, only his ski pole and one of his arms were visible. It took some time to set him free and then start CPR. A long time had passed; perhaps too long.

The situation was dire. The young man had no pulse, and they would have to wait for a rescue; the snow was too deep and unstable to carry out the victim on a pallet. For three hours in the bitter mountainside cold, Gilbert's team pressed ahead with resuscitation efforts. While Gilbert adjusted the breathing tube and pumped the young man's chest, a colleague lit the emergency stove from the camping set and boiled tea to keep them warm. The patient, on the other hand, was kept cold. Every five minutes, the team members would switch places.

When the helicopter was finally able to land, they got the unconscious student up the steep mountainside on a sledge, stumbling through the dark while shivering at the thought of another avalanche. Once on board, they continued CPR, all the while taking care not to raise the patient's temperature. Only after arriving at the hospital did they hook him to a bypass machine to warm him up. Miraculously, the student's heart regained a beat. What's more, his kidneys and lungs had started to function, and his pupils once again shrank in response to light, a sign that his brain was not irreparably damaged. "We were so completely excited," recalls Gilbert. "Very, very, very excited. We thought, 'We finally did it!'"

The young man continued to do well for about two days, but then he took a sudden turn for the worse. In a matter of hours, his brain was crushed by an overload of fluid. In the cramped space of his skull, the pressure was too much, and he died. Gilbert and his team were devastated. They had been so close to a miraculous success, only to have it end the way others had. "I was crazy. I just thought, what did we do wrong? Why were we unable to prevent swelling of the brain?" he said.

As they did after every intensive effort, his team gathered to compare notes on similar cases. Looking back at fifteen similar cases, Gilbert saw that edema, or swelling, was a common problem; the young man had survived longer, but he was not the first to suffer fatal brain swelling after getting back a heartbeat. Gilbert suspected that these half-frozen patients were particularly susceptible. For one thing, hypothermia essentially acts as a blood thinner, so the patients were prone to internal bleeding. But something else was happening that was even more critical. These patients had all suffered cardiac arrest due to hypothermia or been partially suffocated by avalanches or submerged under ice. One way or another, their brains and bodies had been starved of oxygen.

This is where it gets a little tricky and maybe counterintuitive. In effect, these patients were probably all suffering from varying degrees of something known as reperfusion injury. Reperfusion injury is the name for the damage that takes place when oxygen is reintroduced to oxygen-starved tissue. Normally, reintroducing oxygen is good, but with reperfusion injury it seems to set off a complex chain of damaging chemical reactions. The exact mechanism isn't clear, but Gilbert says that cell membranes throughout the body tend to become more permeable—in other words, they start to *leak fluid*—and that is the major cause of swelling.

THE HALF-FROZEN PATIENTS who made it to Tromso were given the standard medications used in resuscitation, such as norepinephrine to stimulate the heart and saline solution to try and maintain normal blood pressure. The problem was, all those infusions meant even more fluid in the body and more pressure on the damaged tissues, including the brain. For Gilbert and his Tromso team, an important and lifesaving lesson had been learned: strictly limit the use of drugs and control the amount of fluid given to a patient in hypothermia, and they are more likely to be saved.

Under normal circumstances, giving fluid to control blood pressure is a staple of emergency medicine, but Gilbert was on to something. He thought this normally lifesaving fluid was also killing his hypothermic patients. "As long as you're a monk, you keep ringing the bell—keep doing the same thing, and you don't look back," he said.

The next time would be different. Gilbert told his team

to forget about the fluids when the next patient came in. They would withhold saline and any other medication unless the patient's clinical condition began to sharply deteriorate. Gilbert said, "On this next one, I'm going to keep it so dry, so restrictive—I'm going to err on the side of not giving fluids unless I'm absolutely forced to."

It was a gamble, but Gilbert was philosophical, saying, "We generate new knowledge and new medical practice in several ways. One is the perspective of controlled clinical trials. Another is taking the problem to the lab, where you do some basic research and then try to apply it." But it was only the third way that could potentially help Anna Bagenholm. That is to *generate* new knowledge through clinical practice.

After landing, Bagenholm was wheeled through the swinging doors of the emergency department and onto an elevator straight to the operating room, where cardiac surgeons ran tubes into Bagenholm's femoral artery and vein and attached her to a heart-lung machine. The machine would slowly rewarm her blood as it maintained circulation. It was approximately 9:50 p.m., and Bagenholm's core body temperature was still just 56 degrees Fahrenheit (13.7 degrees Celsius). As the machine warmed her blood, her heart was still not beating and the team kept up CPR to keep at least some bit of oxygen flowing to her tissues. By 10 p.m., the team saw an encouraging sign. Bagenholm's heart showed a burst of electrical activity on its own. Within another fifteen minutes, the once-still heart had settled into a regular pumping rhythm.

As Gilbert told the story, he paused for a second, then told a story he's not made public before. All of these efforts were nearly derailed by a simple missed detail—that the lifesaving medical team nearly killed their patient that night. While trying to insert a central intravenous line into Bagenholm's chest, a young assistant tore a hole in Bagenholm's subclavian artery. Worse, in the chaos around Bagenholm, no one realized it. Since Bagenholm was virtually dead, her blood pressure was almost nonexistent and there was little blood leaking from the cut.

In a warm, healthy patient such a mistake would be devastating, and the victim would likely bleed to death in minutes. When Bagenholm's heartbeat finally returned, the doctors could see her blood pressure dropping. It was only then that they realized the gravity of the situation. When they put in a chest tube, they watched, horrified, as a full liter of blood poured out. Under pulse-pounding pressure, they raced to open Bagenholm's chest, sawing through bone to find the source of the problem. They were able to suture the artery closed just in time. I couldn't help but marvel at how seemingly simple mishaps like this could derail what would otherwise be striking scientific progress.

As the resuscitation dragged on, Bagenholm developed yet another deadly complication: a breathing problem known as ARDS, in which the lungs are not capable of normal gas exchange. Gilbert's team connected her to a device called ECMO that acts as an artificial lung. She now had a beating heart that produced blood pressure, kidneys that produced urine, and lungs supported by both ventilator and the ECMO-machine. At last they could leave the operating room.

Even then, Gilbert knew they were not out of the woods. "When we took her out of the OR, it was morning. There was sun coming through the windows into the room, and I realized we were in the very same room as the young student," said Gilbert. (The student who had died after the avalanche a few months earlier.) "I said to myself, 'This is not over yet. This is where the struggle starts.'"

This time, the team at Tromso took a more patient approach. They made sure to keep Bagenholm dry (little hydration) and continued to slowly rewarm her. They gave limited drugs and no extra intravenous fluids. For a time, her blood pressure was extremely low, which meant her tissues were not getting as much oxygen as a healthy person requires, but Gilbert guessed that someone in Bagenholm's condition would not need as much oxygen. Otherwise, he reasoned, she could not have survived nearly ninety minutes under the ice.

The road back wasn't easy. For five days Bagenholm remained connected to a machine that helped oxygenate her blood, and she spent another several weeks attached to a respirator, or breathing machine. "She [almost] died two or three times from complications," says Gilbert. "It was a hell of a struggle." But in the end, the all-out effort paid off. A woman who most doctors in the world would have left for dead was alive and breathing, all on her own.

She was paralyzed from the neck down for five months, and yet eighteen months later, Bagenholm was back at work, albeit without full function of her hands, where some of the nerves had been badly damaged. She had to give up being a surgeon, but today she is a full-fledged, successful physician, a radiologist at the University of North Norway Hospital, the same place where she returned from the dead. Interestingly, she says that testing over the years has found that her nerves continue to regrow, ten years after the accident. Her companions from that day work at the same hospital; Marie Falkenberg accomplished her goal of treating children, and Torvind Næsheim now works side by side with Gilbert, riding the ambulance helicopter and aiding in open-heart surgeries as a cardiothoracic anesthesiologist. He has been part of the team that's successfully rewarmed several people in cardiac arrest and with severe hypothermia.

ON THE OTHER side of the world, Zeyad Barazanji was also in need of a doctor who was willing to take a chance. After hearing his story, I went back to the place where his life was truly saved—not the Bronx gym where he collapsed in cardiac arrest and was revived, not the ambulance that raced him to the hospital, but the room where he slowly but surely fought for his life.

While there, I heard a buzzer sounding and a voice calling over the loudspeakers: "Dermatology Floor. Arrest. Stat. Dermatology. Arrest. Stat. Dermatology." The voice is muffled, but the message is urgent: Cardiac arrest. Stat. Dermatology. A patient on another floor has had something go horribly wrong. Her heart has stopped, and it will take all the efforts of modern medicine to keep her from the grave.

If this were a television show, doctors would scramble

down the hall, white coats flying, toward the scene of the emergency. There would be a sense of barely controlled chaos. Here, on the eighth floor of New York-Presbyterian Hospital/Columbia University Medical Center, it barely registers that a life-and-death message is being broadcast through the building.

I am in the neurointensive care unit, an incongruously friendly and easygoing place. A right turn off the elevators, then a left, and without going through a door, you find yourself smack in the middle of a coffee break. The walls are yellow, the floor covered with large square tiles of orange and white. Everything is too new to be coated with the haze of gray that seems to fill most big city hospitals or the grit that permeates the outside of these grand old buildings on the far Upper West Side of New York City.

Nurses talk among themselves at one station, and a group of young people in white coats—mostly men—are huddled, like a football team, around two computer monitors at the other end of the rectangular corridor. Smiles flash, greetings are exchanged, and it takes a few minutes to register what seems to be missing: the patients.

The patients are here, of course, but you could say that's a matter of interpretation. "If you need to be admitted to a neurointensive care unit, it's the worst thing that's ever happened to you in your life," says Dr. Stephan Mayer, the head of the unit. "All of the patients are in varying degrees of coma. For the most part, they're being kept alive artificially."

This morning, a constantly shifting group—a mix of senior physicians, residents in training, and medical students—is huddled around a tiny counter in the middle of the room, framed by two sleek computer monitors. They're staring at a screen displaying data from the Sunrise Clinical Manager, where detailed patient records are stored. Nearly everyone is dressed in a white coat, their specialties etched in blue cursive over the left breast: "Intracranial Monitoring," "Stroke Fellow," "Pediatric Neurology."

The only exception to the dress code is Mayer, who looks like a college freshman in khakis and a blue-and-white striped dress shirt. Small, plain wire-rimmed glasses are perched on his nose, and he quizzes his charges in a friendly, if insistent, slightly nasal voice.

"Can we remember her blood sugar values?"

No answer.

"Come on, people, I'm thinking it's hypoglycemia," he answers quickly himself.

On an especially cold November night in 2006, Mayer took a midnight call from an intense, dark-haired former medical student. He barely knew her; she'd been in the unit the year before, finishing up her rotations. A few months later she had interviewed for a job in the unit, but there was no money to hire her and she ended up in San Francisco. Just the usual comings and goings, but when he took the late-night call he guessed it wasn't to reminisce. When acquaintances called him late at night, they usually had something else on their minds.

On the phone, Nobl Barazangi's[8] voice was friendly but tense. An uncle, an elderly but otherwise healthy man, had suffered a cardiac arrest that afternoon, and he was up in intensive care at another Columbia-affiliated hospital. She didn't trust the doctor running the ICU—mainly because he didn't know anything about hypothermia—and was there an open bed down on 168th Street? "She knew to call here, because she had seen what was happening with the patients here," Mayer told me. "She said, 'Hey, my uncle is thirty-four blocks from you—can you cool him?' And of course I said, 'Sure!'"

When she talks about her uncle that night, Nobl Barazangi focuses on the clinical details, not the stress of being on the other side of the country, desperately seeking help for her father's beloved brother. Though a physician herself, she described the sometimes heart-wrenching difficulty many of us have experienced with elderly parents living far away. She says the first doctor who saw her uncle told her there really wasn't much to be done. "He said they were planning to send him to their intensive care unit for evaluation of his heart, and then just wait for him to either die or wake up," said Barazangi. "I asked if he had considered cooling therapy, and he said he wasn't familiar with it—that he didn't think they did it at his hospital."

It was the middle of the night, and she didn't know exactly what number to call, so she rang up the neurointensive care unit, where she found someone willing to give out Mayer's cell phone number. As she waited on hold, she could feel the seconds ticking away. At the University of California, San Francisco, she had been trained to start cooling patients within an hour of their cardiac arrest. She had learned that with every hour that went by, the odds of survival dropped.

*   *   *

MAYER, TOO, KNEW those statistics well. Mayer is a crusader for therapeutic hypothermia, fretting about doctors who are reluctant to use it as a treatment and the medical organizations who in his view don't do enough to promote it. Mayer first encountered hypothermia in a very different context, on the grounds of an ancient mental hospital in Westchester County, New York. In October 1986, Mayer was a third-year medical student, and he spent most of that month looking after young men who had basically fallen apart under the strain of their freshman year in college. "Depression, bipolar disorder, borderline personality disorder—they were all these young guys who had gone off from home for the first time, and just decompensated under the pressure," he said.

One night, a young man came into the unit in a straitjacket, clearly in the midst of a complete breakdown. "He was in this psychotic rage," says Mayer. "We were giving him doses, megadoses, of Thorazine, Haldol, you name it, and it wasn't touching him at all. He just kept going. And then someone said, 'Get the cold sheets!' And I'm like, 'What's that?' "

Next thing he knew, says Mayer, he was helping more than a dozen doctors and orderlies hold down the unruly patient, while someone else soaked the sheets in ice water and rolled the patient up like a caterpillar in his cocoon. "It was amazing. He immediately calmed down. It worked like nothing else. It was right away. [The young man] said something like, 'Oh, I think I feel okay now.' "

Curious, Mayer asked around and learned that cold

sheets had been widely used in psychiatric hospitals in the early twentieth century.[9] The practice had been widely abandoned, but not by the elderly psychiatrist who ran the institution where Mayer spent that eventful fall. Mayer knew he didn't really understand what he had witnessed, but something about it left a deep imprint.

"I never saw it again, but I was very impressed that something natural and so simple could have such an impact. It was like his brain was boiling with rage, and they just cooled it down," said Mayer. "I thought that for such a natural intervention, it was very powerful." That little lesson would one day set the template for his life's crusade.

A hyperactive teenager who loved new wave bands like Blondie and the Ramones and rambling around the big city with his friends, Mayer was not the most focused student. But he was smart, ambitious, and knew from the first that he wanted to study medicine. The frosty winters were one reason he chose to go to college at Cornell University in frozen Ithaca, New York. Another reason is that he didn't get into his first choice, Yale, or his second choice, Columbia.[10]

He did manage to get into Columbia for medical school and by his senior year was thinking about ways to make his mark. Internal medicine was fine, Mayer told me, "But I thought it might be too vanilla. Part of me wanted to do neurosurgery, but I knew in my heart that I would only be average at best with my hands. There are so many great doctors here. I figured if I did neurosurgery, I would never end up at Columbia—I'd be at some small hospital in the middle of nowhere. But in neurocritical care, I saw an opportunity.

No one was doing it; it was so unexplored. And I got into this field when it was really just being invented."

Mayer got his appointment in the neurology department at Columbia but found he hated it. He felt it was too cerebral; most of the patients were comatose and the treating doctors spent most of their time in academic discussions. Mayer yearned for more action. He wanted to go back to internal medicine. By 1993, however, he discovered a project that would hold his interest. He designed a pilot study testing the safety of hypothermia for patients who had suffered middle cerebral artery infarctions or strokes.

When there is a blockage in the middle cerebral artery, the middle of three major blood vessels bringing blood to the brain, it causes catastrophic brain damage. Here's the problem: as the brain cells, or neurons, start to die from lack of blood flow, the brain starts to swell in response. Swelling in the abdomen and other parts of the body can be serious, but when it pushes the brain against the hard casing of the skull, it's deadly. In any brain injury, swelling and pressure is the biggest threat. Many people got a glimpse of this threat when the actress Natasha Richardson died after falling on a ski slope near Montreal. While the accident seemed minor at first, bleeding inside her head ratcheted up the pressure on Richardson's brain so quickly that within hours of her fall the case was deemed hopeless.[11]

As Mayer embarked on his very first hypothermia study, he wanted to see if therapeutic cooling might reduce the swelling from brain injury, reduce the damage, or both. "Decades ago, the only use of hypothermia was in selected, super-high-risk brain and heart operations, where they needed to completely stop circulation for an extended period of time," says Mayer. This was the legacy of the pioneering heart surgeons. In those early years, hypothermia developed an ominous reputation. While it made daring surgeries possible, patients suffered enough side effects to give doctors serious pause. Patients cooled below 30 degrees Celsius were prone to developing heart arrhythmias. They were also prone to strokes and other types of internal bleeding, since blood that is chilled doesn't clot as well. Most of those early cardiac patients would get better in the short term, but then eventually die of pneumonia. The problem was that in the 1940s, there were no artificial ventilators, so comatose patients had to breathe on their own and their lungs often filled with various secretions. On top of that, hypothermia tends to suppress the immune system, so these patients would develop fatal infections.[12]

But within a few years there were hints and clues that it might be done safely. For example, in 1958 surgeons at the University of Minnesota reported cooling a fifty-one-year-old female cancer patient to just 48 degrees Fahrenheit for her surgery, and rewarming her with no apparent problems.[13] Other experimenters, working with monkeys, also reported good results using extremely low temperatures, and there were even reports of physicians successfully using hypothermia in the treatment of cardiac arrest patients.[14]

By the 1990s, while hypothermia was still out of favor due to safety concerns, Mayer and a few other doctors decided it was time for a fresh look. Mayer suspected that the real problem in the 1940s and 1950s lay not with the cooling itself, but with the follow-up care and nascent level of life-support equipment. He and other doctors felt that some of the pitfalls could be avoided. For one thing, they wouldn't be cooling people to such an extreme degree—they hoped to get results by cooling to around 90 degrees Fahrenheit, not 60 or 70. Just as important, in the modern critical care setting, they could do much better preventing and treating complications like pneumonia.

Over the next decade, Mayer navigated the stepping-stones of an academic career. Along with a handful of other physicians—most notably from Johns Hopkins—he helped to found the first society of neurocritical care specialists and the journal *Neurocritical Care*.[15] And he pushed ahead with studies on hypothermia. One, published in 2001, found that severe stroke patients who were cooled did no worse than uncooled patients.[16] The field of neuroscience, long seen as one where doctors could do little for their patients, was finally shifting and so was that line between life and death.

AS IS USUALLY the case in medical discovery, our best new research is built on existing research. For example, one of the early articles in Mayer's journal was about a discovery that took place when I was still a resident. The Food and Drug Administration (FDA) approved the use of a drug called tissue plasminogen activator, or tPA, to treat patients with strokes.

In one type of stroke, blood flow to part or all of the

brain is cut off by a clot. Without blood flow, that portion of the brain dies. Using tPA is a great option, because it can almost immediately break open the clot and restore blood flow to the brain. The problem is, tPA needs to be given very quickly—within three hours of the start of symptoms—for it to help. For this reason, it's estimated that fewer than 5 percent of stroke patients actually receive this vitally important drug. Enter the Ice Doctor.

A handful of neurologists—Mayer included—thought that hypothermia could be a vital addition to the arsenal. They started experimenting—on the theory that hypothermia would reduce the brain's need for oxygen during the first crucial days of recovery and so reduce the permanent damage. This would reduce the damage caused by lack of oxygen and perhaps extend the window of effectiveness for other therapies, like tPA. Unlike the early cardiac surgeons, Mayer and these other Ice Doctors used a mild form of hypothermia, generally cooling the body by 5 to 10 degrees Fahrenheit.

No doubt, Mayer had cold on the brain, and in 2000, he got more encouragement. A European research team, led by the Austrian emergency medicine specialist Dr. Fritz Sterz, reported that chilling patients by about 7 degrees Fahrenheit was enough to sharply improve the outcome in patients who suffered a life-threatening cardiac arrest.[17] Think about that. Think about the number of times we hear, "He or she died of a heart attack." All the technology in the world's best hospitals could only do so much, but take away 7 degrees Fahrenheit.... When Mayer described all this to me, it seemed counterintuitive that a neurologist would dedicate himself to changing cardiac care around the country. But the Ice Doctor was hooked.

The thing was, Mayer couldn't start cooling cardiac patients on his own simply because he thought it was a good idea. Just because an article gets published doesn't mean its ideas will become accepted practice. That's doubly true if the work is published overseas and even truer in a field like cardiac care, which is so strictly bound by rules and guidelines. In the United States, no one was doing hypothermia. But in Europe, its use continued to grow, and a decade later—medicine moves slowly—there was more ammunition for people like Mayer and for other devotees like the Penn Medicine team led by Lance Becker.

Once again, it came from Sterz' group in Austria, this time under the heading of the Hypothermia After Cardiac Arrest Study Group. The Austrians, led by Dr. Michael Holzer and Sterz, reported in the *New England Journal of Medicine* that they had cooled 136 cardiac arrest patients and 55 percent emerged from the hospital with healthy brain function. In a control group of 137 patients—cardiac arrest victims who were *not* cooled—just 39 percent got better.[18] It wasn't a large study, but it was a strong result published in a major U.S. medical journal. Mayer thought it would be decisive, a triumphant breakthrough, for doctors like him who thought that hypothermia should be the standard treatment.

But that's not how it worked out. With such common and deadly illnesses as heart attacks and strokes, physicians are loathe to experiment—they stick closely to protocol. This is especially true in the United States, where the fear of lawsuits makes doctors especially unwilling to deviate from what might be called the accepted standard of care. For three years after the publication of Fritz Sterz' groundbreaking European study, a handful of American doctors fumed as the American Heart Association (AHA) refused to update its guidelines to require cooling as a treatment for cardiac arrest.

Stephan Mayer was especially steamed. In his view, as long as hypothermia was not considered standard of care, hospitals could rationalize not doing it. After all, if the AHA didn't think it was absolutely necessary, many would ignore it. In 2005, the AHA's guidelines for treating cardiac arrest were rewritten, as they are every five years, and they did list therapeutic hypothermia as a *recommended* treatment—but still not that elusive standard of care.[19]

A key hurdle to shifting that line, once and for all, was the FDA. In 2004, an FDA panel that makes recommendations on medical devices gathered to discuss the evidence for hypothermia and whether companies could specifically market cooling systems for the treatment of cardiac arrest patients. The European study was touted, along with a second study from Australia, which also showed that cooling helped survival.

But things didn't go as Mayer, among many, expected. An influential FDA representative was not swayed by evidence of the benefits from hypothermia. Dr. Julie Swain, a prominent cardiologist, laid into the two studies.[20] She argued that they were too small to suggest a real benefit and pointed to studies of hypothermia in other groups of patients—heart attack victims and people who suffered head injuries—as showing no benefits at all. What's more, she said, patients in those other studies suffered higher rates of side effects like shock and bleeding.

According to Lance Becker, who was at the meeting as an expert consultant, the mood in the room was tense. Becker tried to persuade the panel that hypothermia was worth the risk. Of course the studies were relatively small, he argued, since most cardiac arrest patients die before they even reach the hospital. He pushed on, saying that the two studies together provided more evidence of benefits than existed for many other more accepted therapies. Another consultant, Dr. Joseph Ornato from Virginia Commonwealth University, backed Becker, saying the European and Australian studies were well designed and that it would be wrong—and extremely difficult—to wait for larger studies.

But the enthusiasm had gone out of the room. A third consultant, Dr. John Somberg from Cornell, was blunt. "Forget about their being in the *New England Journal*," he said. "I just do not believe these two studies meet any FDA advisory standard of approval."[21] Somberg, who was a former member of the FDA committee making the decision, went on to compare the two studies to a poorly balanced stack of cards. In the end, his opinion carried the day. Despite the efforts of doctors like Stephan Mayer, hypothermia would not become standard of care.

You may be wondering why I include this losing battle

of the Ice Doctors. Well, herein lies one of the great challenges of medicine. When does an experimental treatment become a standard tool in the doctor's bag? Move too slowly, and you're holding back a treatment that could save thousands of lives. Move too quickly, and you might miss side effects. Look what happened in the case of Vioxx. The FDA approved Vioxx as an antiarthritis medication only to take it off the market five years later, when it became apparent that the drug was linked to heart problems. The FDA says Vioxx probably caused more than 88,000 heart attacks, in all. Maybe they all could have been avoided if the FDA had waited for more evidence before agreeing that the drug was safe.

Critics like Swain and Somberg say the research on hypothermia is thin and, considering the potential risks, not enough to justify its widespread use. But there are major hurdles to actually doing more studies. In a true catch-22, in 2008, the National Institutes of Health (NIH) rejected a proposed study at Duke that would have tested therapeutic cooling against a noncooling regimen, on the grounds that it wouldn't be ethical to withhold cooling.[22] If you think it's confusing—you're right. You've got the FDA saying it's wrong to cool cardiac arrest patients because we don't know if hypothermia works; the AHA saying it's probably a good idea to use the treatment; and the NIH saying the evidence is so strong, it's unethical *not* to cool them.

Whatever the reason, hospitals and doctors in the United States have been slow to adopt the treatment. Medivance, which makes the most widely used therapeutic cooling pads, says that just a few hundred U.S. hospitals—of nearly six thousand total—have even installed the necessary equipment.[23] This sluggish response is especially bewildering, considering the lifesaving success that's taken place in institutions that do adopt the use of cooling. Just one example: after making hypothermia a standard protocol in 2006, the Virginia Commonwealth University Medical Center reported that the death rate for cardiac arrest patients was cut in half.[24]

As I researched this book, I was incredulous that this lifesaving treatment could be ignored by so many. As I described it to my friends and colleagues, they thought it was outrageous. What was the reason? Dr. Raina Merchant, a physician and researcher at the Center for Resuscitation Science, tried to explain. Merchant has conducted a number of studies and surveys, talking to hospitals and doctors about their use of hypothermia and other therapies.[25] She is thirty-one years old, an accomplished physician, but she looks almost like an undergraduate—petite, with studious glasses and often a neat black dress. She is African American, which stands out in the world of leading emergency physicians and cardiologists. I started right into it: why don't more doctors use hypothermia, when the evidence seems to show it's a lifesaver? "At first, we used to think it was because it wasn't in the guidelines," she said. "But now, since 2005, we have that."[26] By this Merchant was talking about the modest recommendation from the American Heart Association.

You might think it costs too much, but according to

Merchant, that's not the problem, either. When I take non-physicians to an ICU and show them the hypothermia equipment, they are always a bit surprised. I think they imagine futuristic ice tubs with bluish solutions coursing through the patient's bloodstream. The truth is, hypothermia is not especially high tech. Doctors pump cool saline through a patient's veins or wrap cold solution-filled pads around the torso and extremities. Picture the opposite of a hot water bottle.

To be fair, the box used to cool and pump the iced slurry solution costs about $25,000. But even if $25,000 sounds like a lot of money, when compared to therapies like dialysis, it's cheap. Cost-benefit studies showed the box would actually save money. Merchant told me, "If you cool even one patient and avoid complications, you save more than the cost of dozens of boxes. It's cheaper to cool than not to cool." And even the box isn't absolutely necessary. Ice bags will do the trick, although it's harder to control the temperature. According to Lance Becker, for years, heart surgeons in Russia would pack a patient's chest cavity with ice until it was cold enough to stop the heart. Fritz Sterz, the Austrian physician who pioneered the use of hypothermia in Europe, tells of a case where he used bags of frozen vegetables from a grocery freezer to cool a patient who had collapsed in a grocery aisle.

In other words, it is a recommended, rather cost-effective therapy. I had to ask: "What am I missing here?" In Merchant's view, the biggest hurdle to widespread use of hypothermia is a psychological one. Her colleague in the

University of Pennsylvania emergency department, Dr. Ben Abella, explained, "It's a paradigm shift. We're using this for people whose eyes are yellow, they're not moving, and you're telling doctors to cool these people for twenty-four hours—then warm them up for a day, then take them to the cath lab. You're doing all these things for people who look dead, sound dead, and act dead. It's asking a lot."

Abella sees a parallel to the resistance that met the first groundbreaking chemotherapy treatments in the 1930s. At that time, cancer was a truly hopeless diagnosis, and many doctors were defeatist about it. "There was a certain sense of 'everyone is going to die, so why waste all this money and time?'" he said.

It may be that lack of hope leads to inertia and apathy, but as I dug deeper, I found even more reasons therapeutic hypothermia has been slow to catch on. Here's one that will probably make you angry: using hypothermia might be inexpensive and effective, but it isn't nearly as simple as rolling out a new miracle drug. In this case, being inexpensive is not necessarily an asset, but a potential liability. For example, let's say you've invented this new medication. You run studies comparing the new pill to a placebo, publish the results, and then—assuming it works—you send the sales team to tell physicians about it. If they're convinced, the doctors start writing prescriptions. There is no doubt money to be made.

By contrast, a single doctor, no matter how motivated, can't just start writing prescriptions for hypothermia. He or she has to convince a hospital to buy the equipment; it might not be terribly expensive as medical equipment goes, but it's enough that a purchasing committee needs to get involved. It gets even more complicated. A cardiac arrest patient is as likely to be treated as a neurology patient as a cardiology patient, and in either case, he or she almost certainly starts in the emergency department. All three of those departments have to not only agree that hypothermia is useful, they have to agree on where to get the money to buy the gear. Then they have to figure out a protocol for identifying patients who would be helped by the treatment—and train people to do it properly. This would be hard enough in a single hospital department; with two or three departments involved, it can be a bit like herding cats. Even a good idea, without the millions of dollars that are often backing a new drug, has a hard time getting off the ground. There is a sometimes ugly underbelly of medical progress, and this is just one example of it.

On the Penn Medicine website, Becker and his colleagues have posted the hypothermia protocols from more than two dozen medical centers.[27] There's no special qualification; someone just has to be willing to e-mail their institution's guidelines. Since setting up the website, the Center for Resuscitation Science has received thousands of e-mails from hospitals who want to set up their own hypothermia programs. The hope is that by making the details easily and publicly available, Becker and his team will inspire others to start—and will take away the excuse that hypothermia programs are all too complicated.

Raina Merchant found that the most common reason

hospitals start using hypothermia is because there's a doctor or even a nurse who knows about hypothermia and talks it up among their colleagues. If there's no local champion, no one gets cooled. Like a lot of things in medicine, it boils down to word of mouth, the squeaky wheel. Simply put, despite all the technology and years of studies, hypothermia still needs champions like Stephan Mayer.

At Columbia, when it comes to hypothermia, it's full speed ahead. After receiving the midnight call from Nobl Barazangi, Mayer called the hospital that was treating her uncle and arranged a transfer. Thirty minutes later, Zeyad Barazanji was in Mayer's ICU, being strapped to the cooling pads and blankets.[28] His temperature was falling. Mayer could only hope that it would hold down the chaos bubbling up in the professor's wounded, oxygen-deprived brain cells.

Watching over Barazanji was a nurse, Mary Grace Savage, who had her own story to tell. That spring, her husband, a senior official with the New York Fire Department, suffered a cardiac arrest at his gym in Brooklyn. Two fellow firefighters performed CPR to get his heart going again, but he was still unconscious when he was taken to the local hospital. When Savage found out, she had him transferred to Columbia immediately. She believes that if it had been just another hour or two longer, he might not have made it. As it is, he was out of the hospital in eight days and back at work within six months.[29]

As these success stories start to percolate, the tide has lately been turning. In early 2009, the New York

Fire Department announced bold new plans to cool cardiac arrest patients in the field, and to only take them to hospitals that practice cooling. "The plan is to make therapeutic hypothermia the first thing out of the bag, right after defibrillation," says FDNY Medical Director John Freese. "Once we get the breathing tube and an IV placed, we'll just give everyone two liters of cooled saline."[30]

In preparation, Freese has had to identify which hospitals are able to efficiently cool patients coming in from the field. After all, it would make no sense to cool a cardiac arrest victim in their home, only to let them warm up thirty minutes later when they reach the hospital. The process has not been tension free. There was shouting at one meeting, when the head of a major hospital group said he didn't want to publicly compare survival rates at different hospitals—it might embarrass someone. Similar efforts are underway in Arizona, Wisconsin, and Seattle.

Lance Becker insists that doubters are missing the forest for the trees; whatever side effects exist are minimal in contrast to the life-preserving power of cold. "No matter which direction you go, whether you're conservative or aggressive, we know it will save people's lives," said Becker. "How many lives have been lost, because we delayed implementing this for a year or two? I have to think that we've lost lives, because we've failed to move aggressively."

The practice of medicine is changing constantly. The innovation isn't always for the better—ask one of the women who took thalidomide in the 1960s to ward off morning sickness. And innovation is never easy—most of the first heart transplant patients died within hours or days of their transplant. But the next round of transplants went better, and then better, and today thousands of heart transplant patients live rich lives because of the bold pioneers of the 1950s and 1960s and their brave subjects. What I have learned is that this cycle—desperation, desperate measure, apparent miracle, insight, common practice—shifts the line in the sand. That's how medicine moves forward. When Mads Gilbert saw his lifeless, near-frozen patient, what if he had thrown his hands in the air, and said, "We've done all we can do"? Would he have been unreasonable?

Hypothermia is no antidote to death, no cure for cardiac arrest. What it does is buy time. Today, minutes, or hours, but some scientists have more dramatic goals. The European Space Agency, the counterpart to NASA, reportedly has studied extreme hypothermia—cryonics—as a way to preserve astronauts for distant journeys through the solar system, trips too long to bring sufficient food or water. Some people say extended preservation using extreme cold could someday be part of routine medical care. The British futurist Aubrey de Grey, whose scientific foundation is seeking ways to radically increase longevity, predicts that in the future virtually any ailment will be reversible, anything short of total physical destruction.[31] The trick is to somehow preserve our bodies until such technology exists. Grey says cryonics is an extremely promising technique: "This is not bringing people back from the dead. This is a form of critical care."

Cryonics is already starting to find its way into the

lay public. At least two private companies, including the Arizona-based Alcor Life Extension Foundation, are already using cryonics to preserve paying customers at extremely low temperatures. Alcor says that its process— called vitrification—uses organ preservation fluid that enables rapid cooling without creating ice crystals that would damage individual cells. The bodies are stored in gleaming metal tanks at the bottom of a bubbling pool of liquid nitrogen; it looks like water, but it's no hot tub: the temperature is minus-196 degrees Celsius. Despite a price tag of $150,000 (with a bargain rate of $80,000 for neuro-preservation—i.e., just having your head frozen), Alcor says it has already chilled more than eighty people and signed up nearly nine hundred members to follow in their footsteps.[32] Lest it be seen as an out-of-reach luxury, Alcor Executive Director Jennifer Chapman notes that most customers pay using proceeds of their life insurance.

According to Alcor's website, cryonic preservation needs to begin within fifteen minutes of the heart stopping, and ideally within just a minute or two. Otherwise, too much damage is done to cells in the process of death. Along those same lines, Mads Gilbert believes it was the suddenness of Anna Bagenholm's plunge through the ice that may have saved her. "If you're suffocated while you're still warm, it's like hanging or drowning," he explains. "You can probably forget it."

That pessimism largely stems from an experience Gilbert had in 1989, helping to rescue Norwegian soldiers trapped in an avalanche during NATO's winter training exercise: thirty-one troops were trapped; sixteen of them died—most from hypothermia, as their body temperature *slowly* dropped inside their snowy prison. It is true that as the body cools, every organ needs less oxygen. But when that cooling process is dragged out, it means an extended time where oxygen demand is high, even as supply—the ability to breathe—stays low. That means irreversible damage. Had the soldiers fallen into frozen water causing a sudden and dramatic drop in body temperature, says Gilbert, it could have turned out differently. "If you fall in through the ice, you're cool before you even stop breathing," he said. "That's Anna."

Bagenholm herself remembers nothing of the accident, only waking up to find herself in critical care. In an interview a year later, she said she's as surprised as anyone to still be here. "When you're a patient, you're not thinking you are going to die. You think, I'm going to make it," said Bagenholm. "But as a medical person, I think it's amazing that I'm alive."[33]

She told my team she never despaired, even in the darkest days when she was still paralyzed in intensive care. "As a doctor, I understood a lot of things that were happening. I knew there was no spinal cord damage. I just waited to see what would happen. I focused on slowly getting better, trying do to the things I could. I never thought about not going back to work."

Gilbert maintains that the rescue was no miracle: "It's the simple things, not the complicated things." Success came not from any high-tech solution, but from fifteen years of hard work and intuition honed by trial and error. "It was the whole system, from the way we interact with local resources to the way we include the hospital at the end," said Gilbert. "We'd had mistakes with other patients. We nearly succeeded, but lost them. By the time Anna came in, we'd adjusted some of the treatment. . . . The team on call that very night was a very well-geared team, tightly woven, with a strong spirit and optimism."

Bagenholm still goes hiking and skiing on a near daily basis. She and Gilbert are friends. In fact, the day he finally shared the full details of Bagenholm's case, he had just spent the weekend with her and a close friend, skiing on the same slopes that sparked the frustration and inspiration for his most famous rescue.

CHAPTER TWO

A Heart-Stopping Moment

And he went up, and lay upon the child, and put his mouth upon his mouth, and his eyes upon his eyes, and his hands upon his hands: and stretched himself upon the child; and the flesh of the child waxed warm.

—2 Kings 4:34, KJV

MIKE MERTZ WAS driving home, an hour after finishing his run as a school bus driver in Glendale, Arizona. He told me he doesn't remember why he didn't come straight home from work that day. He thinks that maybe he went for a jog. A trim fifty-nine years old, Mertz enjoyed a two- or three-mile run several days a week. Maybe he was looking for a cheaper gas station than the one on his usual route or was just trying to avoid taking his Saturn over a nasty set of new speed bumps. Whatever the reason, whatever route he wandered, it brought Mertz not to the usual entrance of his townhome complex, but the back driveway.[1] The change in routine may have saved his life.

Corey Ash, a UPS driver, was making deliveries that Wednesday afternoon, when he heard a terrible engine noise. Thinking the sound was underneath his own hood, he pulled over. Hopping out, Ash immediately realized that it was coming from a Saturn almost directly across the street.

It was an accident scene. The small silver car was piled up against a palm tree, the engine revving at top speed. The only thing keeping it in place was a stucco wall a few feet from the tree; the car was wedged between the two. Racing over, Ash could see that the driver had his eyes closed and seemed to be unconscious. The driver's foot was wedged against the accelerator. Ignoring the chance that the car might break free and crush him, Ash reached across the slumped body and turned off the ignition. He dragged Mertz out of the car and laid him on the ground. After dialing 911, Ash started CPR the way he'd learned during an Air National Guard training exercise just two months before.

As he listened to the ambulance siren, racing up the road from Glendale Fire Station 154 barely a mile away, Ash began to pump hard on Mertz' chest. Studies show that when a bystander jumps in, the chances of survival in a cardiac arrest case increase exponentially. Even though it may not seem like you are accomplishing much, simply pushing the heart and circulating the blood can make a tremendous difference. Mertz had that going for him, but he was also fortunate to have collapsed in Glendale. Paramedics there are at the forefront of a revolution in emergency care. With a few simple measures—going against the grain of the medical establishment—they have found that they can radically improve the odds of surviving a cardiac arrest.

The fire engine pulled up with a screech, and a brawny firefighter named Ruben Florez jumped to the curb. As fellow firefighters scrambled down, Florez thumped an urgent rhythm on Mertz' chest, two hundred compressions over two minutes, before a medic stepped in and delivered an electric shock from the paddles of a defibrillator.

Then came another two hundred compressions, then shock, two hundred compressions, then shock. Finally, after six hundred thumps and three defibrillator shocks, a weak pulse returned. Mertz was back from the dead. At no point was mouth-to-mouth resuscitation performed, and at no point did Mike Mertz get a breath. Surprisingly, that may be the *real reason* he survived.

In reality, survival from cardiac arrest outside the hospital is rare. Until very recently, Arizona was in line with the rest of the country—only about 2 percent of the victims pulled through without long-term damage.[2] But in 2005, cities around Arizona began doing something new. It went against the guidelines of the American Medical Association and the teaching practices of major medical schools and hospitals. This new method didn't look like the CPR that had been taught in every YMCA, firehouse, school, and church ever since the 1970s. In short, it was a radical experiment.

The experiment sprang from two lines of thinking: animal studies aimed at modifying CPR technique and a public health effort to train more people in CPR. If your heart gives out while you're walking down the street, the number-one thing that can save your life is to have a bystander who is not only trained in CPR, but willing to help. Unfortunately, such help is rare. Published studies put the rate of bystander CPR at around 20 percent.[3] If you dig deep, the number really has nothing to do with the lack of desire. Instead, study after study shows people are apprehensive about putting their mouth on someone else's and maybe catching an infection from someone who's on the ground dying.

Now, the reluctance can be overcome. In Seattle, which has run massive training programs and public education campaigns since the 1970s, the rate of CPR assistance from bystanders is close to 50 percent.[4] That one fact gets much of the credit for the city's high survival rate from cardiac arrest. In recent years, a driving goal of the American Heart Association has been to encourage more members of the public to jump in and help. But how? There was simply no getting around mouth-to-mouth resuscitation. Or was there?

Cardiologist Dr. Gordon Ewy, and his team at the Sarver Heart Center in Tucson, had been doing CPR experiments for more than twenty years. Their focus was to try to understand the role that artificial breathing plays in emergency resuscitation, and for more than a decade, much to the consternation of the powers that be, Ewy had argued that breathing was nearly irrelevant.

Ewy is cantankerous and opinionated, and he's sure those opinions are right. In other words, he's like a lot of heavyweights in academic medicine. In professional stature, Ewy is decidedly a heavyweight, even if his office is thousands of miles from any ivy-covered wall. After graduating from the University of Kansas, he completed a medical residency at Georgetown. After finishing his training in Washington, D.C., in 1971, Ewy headed west to help launch the University of Arizona's new teaching hospital in Tucson. He's run the cardiology department since 1990, which makes him the longest-serving chief of cardiology in the United States.[5]

Ewy first got interested in CPR research as a way to fine-tune guidelines for the public. For years, studies have shown that people are much more willing to do a simplified version of CPR—if you tell them to stick with chest compressions and don't worry about the mouth-to-mouth part. To Ewy, that itself was more than enough reason to support a change in guidelines. But as he took a closer look at the data, to make sure a modified technique would still be reasonably effective, Ewy started to notice something else, something strange. The survival rates for people getting chest compressions alone weren't only as good as people getting full AHA-approved CPR, they were better. Almost by accident, the public health campaign had stumbled onto a medical discovery.

To understand Ewy's theory about CPR, you have to know about the three-phase model of cardiac arrest, developed by our friend Dr. Lance Becker from the University of Pennsylvania's Center for Resuscitation Science and Myron Weisfeldt of Johns Hopkins University.[6] The three distinct phases are electrical, circulatory, and metabolic. The first lasts approximately four minutes, during which time the heart still pulsates with its own electrical energy, even as it fails to generate a coherent, blood-pumping rhythm. The ensuing circulatory phase lasts from approximately four minutes after cardiac arrest until the ten-minute mark. Whatever oxygen was present in the blood has been consumed, and without oxygen, the heart can no longer generate electrical energy. The absence of oxygen also triggers dangerous chemical reactions throughout the body, as cells turn to sources of stored energy. At a certain point—about ten minutes after cardiac arrest, assuming there is no intervention—the cascade of cell-killing chemical reactions reaches a crescendo. This marks the third step toward death, the metabolic phase. It's during this time that cell death begins in earnest.

The model helps explain why some interventions do work. During the electrical phase, defibrillation is highly effective; after that, not so much. That's because defibrillation doesn't restore electricity to the heart; it just resets the rhythm. For it to work, the heart needs to have enough energy present to resume beating once given the chance, like a car battery with enough juice to still take a jump. No matter how hard you try, you can't restart a completely dead battery.

When you perform CPR, you are in effect sending oxygenated blood to the heart tissue—sort of like kindling to catch the electrical flame of a defibrillator. In traditional CPR, bystanders and paramedics alike are trained to start by checking to see that the airway is clear and to alternate compressions with rescue breaths—mouth to mouth. Paramedics are trained to insert a breathing tube, as well. The artificial breaths are supposed to add oxygen to the blood, and chest compressions are meant to circulate that oxygen. What Ewy realized is that some of that effort might be wasted. From the three-phase model, we see that when breathing ceases, for several minutes there is still a good amount of oxygen sitting in the bloodstream. The human body stores far more oxygen than we are generally aware of, and that oxygen lingers for some time after we've actually stopped breathing. Therein lies an important lesson that turns conventional CPR on its head: maybe, just maybe, those artificial breaths aren't necessary.

The thing is, in order to help, that oxygen has to circulate in the blood. If your heart has stopped, the oxygen can only circulate if someone pumps the heart artificially, by compressing the chest. When you pause to give an artificial breath, you're not pressing on the chest. The same goes for inserting a breathing tube, a sometimes awkward process that usually takes anywhere from twenty to thirty seconds.[7] Even after administering a shock, you're supposed to wait and read the heart rhythm, to see if the shock has worked—and try again, if needed. All these extra steps, says Ewy, waste time. Precious time that has cost too many lives.

You don't need the three-phase model to understand that time is at a desperate premium after cardiac arrest. Every second is critical. According to the American Heart Association, for every minute that goes by without someone attempting CPR or defibrillation, the odds of survival decrease by 7 to 10 percent.[8] If ten minutes go by, survival is a long shot. Delay means more than just a lower chance of survival. Every moment without oxygen increases the chance of brain damage should the victim survive. The heart itself is also at risk; as cardiologists like to say, "Time is muscle," heart muscle. Even if a patient survives with brain function nearly intact, extra minutes without oxygen means more dead heart tissue, increasing the severity of cardiovascular disease and the risk of a future heart attack.

In Ewy's view, getting blood and oxygen moving— compressing the chest—is virtually the only thing that matters. In theory, all the extra steps and equipment are lifesaving, but Ewy felt they could just as easily be distractions. In fact, when the city of Seattle initially put defibrillators on their ambulances, survival rates for cardiac arrest actually went down.[9] It's not because defibrillators are a bad idea, just the opposite. But anything that slows down the process of CPR poses a new challenge. "If you stop for anything, it's a disaster," Ewy likes to say.

With a mix of admiration and exasperation, Dr. Ben Abella, who works with Becker as research director at the Center for Resuscitation Science, calls Ewy a zealot for chest compressions. It's an accurate description. The take-away message from Ewy is if you see someone fall to the ground after a cardiac arrest, just start pushing on the chest as fast as you can. To emphasize the goal of preserving full brain function, he dubbed the method CCR, for cardio-cerebral resuscitation.

In the lab, the Sarver team, led by Ewy and cardiologist Dr. Karl Kern, did controlled experiments with animals.

In 1993, they compared research subjects who received only chest compressions during resuscitation from cardiac arrest to subjects who received artificial breaths along with the compressions. The animals who got only compressions didn't just do as well, they did better.[10] After publishing those startling findings, the team kept plugging along. Between 1993 and 2002, they conducted six more studies with pigs, comparing CCR (chest compressions only) to CPR with artificial breaths. They all found the same thing: the breaths provided no extra benefit.[11]

If Ewy's results had been accepted at that time, I probably would have learned a very different sort of CPR when I was in medical school, but there were admittedly a couple of hurdles still to cross. The first problem was, the research subjects were swine, and no one was paying much attention to doctors trying to revive a bunch of pigs. Another problem was that other researchers tried similar experiments and got different results. Their pigs died.[12] When we asked Ewy about that, he was ready with an answer. He says these other studies failed because researchers paralyzed the pigs' chest muscles, so they couldn't gasp in at least a small amount of oxygen during cardiac arrest, as would happen during a "real-world" arrest.

Some doctors still argued that the studies were misleading. One argument that caught my eye was that a pig's trachea, or windpipe, is shaped differently than a human's. But Ewy says critics were setting the bar impossibly high. "When you're talking about cardiac arrest, you just cannot do randomized, controlled trials in people," he told me.

Research on swine, he argues, is a good substitute. "In our animal model, we've come up with a lot of different ways of doing CPR that improve survival in man."

Ewy wanted the American Heart Association to stop telling people to give mouth-to-mouth resuscitation, but for a long time, the AHA didn't see things his way. When it comes to writing guidelines, the AHA lists six criteria that it will consider: Number one, the gold standard, is a randomized, controlled study involving people. Number six is animal studies. To start changing minds, Ewy and his colleagues needed a real-life experiment. But how? Who would possibly be willing to buck the guidance of the national medical organizations? What they needed was someone outside the establishment, someone willing to take a leap of faith.

And then in November 2002, opportunity knocked, more or less out of nowhere. A week after announcing their desire to break with AHA guidelines, Ewy and Kern were at the American Heart Association meeting in Chicago. As always, the meeting was a big one, a virtual small city at the glass-enclosed McCormick Place convention center. Neither of the Arizona physicians had ever seen the burly, bespectacled doctor who strode up out of the crowd.

He introduced himself as Mike Kellum, an ER doctor from southern Wisconsin, just a two-hour drive from the meeting. For almost a decade, he had been the emergency services director for Mercy Health System, a group of clinics and small hospitals serving Rock and Walworth counties. Kellum didn't work in academia, but he liked to read medical journals in his spare time. He had the energy of a young man, but he was nearly sixty, and his keen interest in resuscitation research dated back to the 1980s, when he'd read an article about dogs who were successfully revived after flatlining on a heart monitor for several minutes.[13]

Kellum was well aware that most times when his paramedics were called to the scene of a cardiac arrest, they couldn't offer much help. To me, he described a sense of impotence as EMS director, going through case report after case report: "Looking at these cardiac arrests, reviewing these, you're seeing 'they're dead,' 'they're dead,' one after another. 'Dead, dead, dead, dead.' After all this time, why are we spending time trying to bring *no one* back to life?"

The reports out of Arizona gave Kellum a sense that he might have a way to change the game. In the hallway outside the AHA meeting, he told Ewy that he wanted to see if the new protocol could work among the flat, sprawling dairy farms of southern Wisconsin. Soon after, he flew to Tucson, accompanied by three other EMS directors from Wisconsin. This small group of unknown physicians was launching a major challenge to the field of emergency medicine.

While not a prestigious academic center, Mercy Health System is the dominant medical provider in Rock and Walworth counties, about an hour south of Madison. Its sixty-three facilities handle more than 85,000 patients a year.[14] Kellum's ambulance squads have a lot of ground to cover. Even with sirens blaring full tilt, it takes an ambulance twenty minutes to get from Mercy's main hospital in Janesville to the far western edge of Rock County.[15]

In the three years prior to Kellum's experiment, emergency teams had responded to ninety-two cases of witnessed cardiac arrest. Of those patients, only nineteen survived—and only fourteen without serious brain damage. It was, as Kellum's team wrote in a subsequent paper, an awful record—but no worse, probably better in fact, than the results from the rest of the country. Put bluntly, under the accepted standard of care, the vast majority of patients died.[16]

Once home Kellum and the other EMS directors made a radical decision to change the way they responded to cardiac emergencies. They would try the resuscitation method that had formally been tested, at that point, only on pigs. They would teach it to their paramedics, firefighters and police officers—everyone who was part of the counties' 911 emergency response system. The single focus would be ensuring circulation to the brain. Every effort would focus on chest compressions, and interruptions would be kept to a minimum. When they first came to a patient who had stopped breathing, they would immediately begin by giving not fifteen, not thirty, but two hundred hard and fast compressions to the chest. Emergency responders would follow that with a single shock from a defibrillator rather than the multiple shocks that were considered standard medical procedure.

Defibrillation is a powerful lifesaving tool, but Kellum knew that each shock takes precious time. So after each single shock, emergency responders would give another two hundred chest compressions. Rescue breaths were eliminated entirely. A small device would be inserted into the mouth to pump in additional oxygen, but no breathing tube would be inserted until the patient had a pulse or until he or she had received three rounds of shocks and compressions—six hundred chest compressions in all.

All through 2004, Kellum called down to Tucson with updates. Everything was going great; it was obvious the new technique was working. Paramedics were getting saves they had never gotten before. Ewy was thrilled, but it wasn't enough. He needed other people to know about the results, so every time he got Kellum on the phone, he would harangue him to submit them to an academic journal. Bouncing in his seat across from me, Ewy reenacted the phone calls. "I'd say, 'Mike, you gotta get some data!' After he'd called me up several times, I'd be screaming at him, 'You gotta get some data!' He'd say, 'I'm just an ER doc; I can't do that.' But eventually I just wore him down," said Ewy.

In the fall of 2006, when Kellum finally published his article (Ewy was a coauthor) in the *American Journal of Medicine*, the results were astounding. In the previous three years, of ninety-two people in Rock and Walworth counties who suffered out-of-hospital cardiac arrest, only 15 percent had survived with intact brain function. After the new protocol was implemented, that rate more than tripled. In thirty-three cases of sudden cardiac arrest, nineteen people survived and sixteen of them—48 percent—walked out of the hospital, more or less as good as new. Ewy recalls, "We had a dickens of a time getting it published. People thought this was just too good to believe." But a longer follow-up study found nearly identical results,[17] and in the meantime, Ewy had found a bigger stage to test the theory.

He had also found an important ally, Dr. Bentley Bobrow. Bobrow is a serious, small, almost dainty man in his mid-thirties. As director of emergency services for the state of Arizona, he oversees the training of paramedics, and by 2005, he was familiar with Ewy's research, not to mention the real-life experiments in Tucson and southern Wisconsin. Bobrow decided it was time to try the experiment on a larger scale.

Unlike Gordon Ewy, Bobrow tends to worry out loud—especially about whether a reporter will paint him as a rebel. While Ewy has been described as "a constant thorn in the side of the AHA," Bobrow likes to emphasize what he shares with mainstream thinking. "I don't want to tell anyone else what to do," he says. Still, despite the diplomatic language, the crew cut, the neat white dress shirt and tie, an independent streak sticks out, and not just in medicine. Along with his wife and young son, for example, Bobrow doesn't own a television set.[18] And he doesn't mince words.

"Some people felt it was negligent to not follow the existing guidelines, but if with the guidelines 97 percent of everyone died, we felt it was incumbent on us to try something new" is how Bobrow explains the urgency. But "something new" was a hard sell. In most Arizona cities, emergency response is handled by the fire department. As Bobrow drove from firehouse to firehouse, he got an earful from medics and firefighters who had been doing things the same way for more than two decades. There were paramedics on the job who had been part of Glendale's first-ever CPR class back in the 1970s, when CPR was new and almost miraculous in its promise. The paramedics thought of themselves as medical professionals, and now they weren't supposed to give breaths? *Anyone* could do this?[19]

Patiently, stop after stop, again and again, Bobrow made the pitch. He kept coming back to the same point: What was there to lose? When 97 percent of the patients died, how could they do worse?

In fact, Bobrow and Ewy were confident they would do much better. They'd both heard too many stories to be convinced otherwise. Ewy's favorite one dates back to the mid-1990s when an emergency physician from Seattle played a tape recording for him. It was of a phone call from a woman who called 911 after her husband collapsed and stopped breathing. While an ambulance raced toward the house, the 911 dispatcher tried to guide the woman through basic CPR. The advice would sound familiar to anyone who has taken a CPR class in the past thirty years: Feel for a pulse. Tilt the head back. Check the airway. Listen for breathing. Pinch the nose. Breath into the mouth twice. Fifteen chest compressions. Repeat.

Frightening as the scene must have been, Ewy can't stop grinning when he tells the story. The frantic woman would ask how far away the ambulance was, and the dispatcher would send her back to continue CPR. "After a while," says Ewy, "she came back to the phone and said, 'Why is it, every time I press on his chest, he opens his eyes, and every time I stop and breathe for him, he goes back to sleep?'" He paused and gave a rueful laugh. "This woman in ten minutes learned more about cerebral perfusion [getting blood flow to the brain] than we had in fifteen or twenty years of CPR research." All that research, Ewy says, points to one thing: "You don't stop pressing on the chest for anything."

By March 2007, Bobrow's firefighters were ready to pull up the curtain on their experiment. The results were better than anyone, except perhaps Ewy, had dreamed. Among all victims of out-of-hospital cardiac arrest, the survival rate more than tripled. Among those whose heart stopped in front of a witness who called 911, it nearly quadrupled. Bobrow set the bar high: he didn't count people as survivors unless they walked out of the hospital without significant brain damage. And yet, among victims of an illness that typically kills more than 95 percent of those it strikes, one in four was walking around almost as if nothing had happened.[20]

As we came to learn, this phenomenon wasn't isolated to small towns in Wisconsin and Arizona. In 2007, researchers in Japan unveiled the results of a massive study on bystander interventions. They examined cases where a person collapsed of sudden cardiac arrest outside of a hospital but in view of a bystander: of those receiving no help before an ambulance arrived, only 3 percent survived; of those who got traditional mouth-to-mouth resuscitation along with chest compressions, the survival rate jumped to 11 percent; but of those who got chest compressions only, it was even better—19 percent.[21]

Kellum says that when he first started telling people about his results, he was met with stark disbelief. At one point, he flew to Kansas City to give a presentation about CCR to a medical group. Afterward, Kellum says, "The top three people went out to dinner and said, 'That guy is certifiably insane.' And then they began to look at the data, and you just can't argue with it."

By tripling the survival rate from cardiac arrest in Arizona, Bobrow estimates his paramedics saved several hundred lives during the three-year study period alone. A medicine that did the same would be a best seller. "It's a phenomenal thing," Bobrow told me. "Here you have a situation where not one nickel has been spent teaching this, and it turns out to be just as good—or in my view, better— than something on which millions of dollars and man-hours have been spent."

In the world of medicine, paradoxically, it can be much harder to convince people to try a simple and inexpensive solution than one that is complex and unproven. Here's my own theory: There are thousands of medical journals churning out new articles every week. Sorting the useful from the useless is a herculean task. Meanwhile, there are approximately 800,000 physicians in the United States, most of whom aren't leafing through medical journals in their spare time. In that sea of information, a new idea or therapy, even one that's a proven success, has to struggle to capture attention. A company with a new wonder drug is often willing to spend millions or even billions of dollars to tell physicians about its benefits. On the other hand, something as basic as a new kind of CPR—well, who's got a stake in that?[22]

ON A FEBRUARY day in 2008, in the mellow afternoon glow of the Arizona winter, Mike Mertz grinned from ear to ear as he walked into Glendale Fire Station 154. He wanted to shake hands with Ruben Florez and the rest of the crew that saved his life. Bentley Bobrow was there, too, shaking his head: "He truly was dead, and here he is, fine."

In medicine, there's often a choice between pursuing the known course, the comfortable course, the well-worn path—and trying something new. Innovation might save lives and yet at the same time cost lives. Medicine in general is geared toward caution. First, do no harm. And yet, our greatest learning comes *not* from never failing, but in learning from our mistakes, rising up every time we do fail.

The smiles lasted a few minutes, until a call came in and Florez and the engine had to pull out. Afterward, in the quiet outside the station, Mertz wondered aloud at the other path he might have taken. When he came in to the hospital, doctors had told his daughter that he most likely wasn't going to make it. "I was completely out. Gone," he said. "If that UPS guy hadn't come around the corner, I wouldn't be here today. It was that close."

Even more than that, if it weren't for the persistent efforts of brave physicians like Gordon Ewy, Mike Mertz probably wouldn't be standing there outside the fire station. He wouldn't have a newly implanted defibrillator, and he wouldn't be looking forward to getting back on the golf course. Just six weeks after he died, the only lingering effect is a set of sore ribs.

Mertz probably owes his life to a handful of physicians who were willing to challenge the rules, if not quite break them. And when the doctors say there was nothing to lose, they have a point. Basic artificial respiration has been around since the 1700s, and the modern technique has been in use for half a century. But a dirty little secret remains: most of the time, it doesn't work. In most cities, "survival to good outcome" for cardiac arrest outside the hospital is still around 2 percent, and in some places, it's even worse. In Detroit during a six-month period in 2002, paramedics responded to more than four hundred cardiac arrest cases and emerged with just a single success story—one patient who survived long enough to make it out of the hospital.[23]

Yet other places seem to have cracked the code. Arizona tripled the survival rate of cardiac arrests. Seattle, with its high percentage of trained bystanders and tradition of innovation in emergency medicine, reports a survival rate of close to 20 percent—and nearly 40 percent in cases where paramedics find a patient whose heart is in ventricular fibrillation, the most "survivable" rhythm.[24] Like Arizona, Seattle now uses a resuscitation method that emphasizes chest compressions. Seattle does something else that's interesting; officials take care not to hire too *many* EMTs. They've found that when they hired too many people, each EMT got less practice and survival rates dropped.[25]

None of this is rocket science or brain surgery. The closer you look, the more you see that it doesn't always require a fancy breakthrough to save tens of thousands of lives. When it comes to cheating death, it sometimes happens that simple measures are more important than the hoops and frills of high-tech medicine. Sometimes a sea change in the world of medicine can be accomplished by lucky accident and the efforts of a few individuals who refuse to accept the conventional wisdom.

CHAPTER THREE

Suspend Disbelief

When does death really take place? I would argue that we don't really know the answer.

—Dr. Lance Becker

A SOLDIER FALLS IN a gully, off a long mountain pass near Khost, Afghanistan, after being hit by sniper fire. His comrades scatter for cover, scanning the hillsides for the sniper. Seeing no target, they let loose with a heavy machine gun to provide cover while a medic tries to reach the fallen man. There's no panic, but there is urgency. The medic tears through his pack, fingers pulling apart the edges of a small syringe. With heavy breaths, he counts off, "One, two, three..." then races across the open ground while his friends lay a withering burst of fire in the general direction of the sniper's position.

When the corporal reaches the fallen man, he feels for a pulse, but the one he finds is so weak that he knows it won't last more than a few minutes. The platoon is dozens of miles from help, and even a helicopter couldn't arrive in time to save the injured soldier. Gritting his teeth, the medic saws open the unconscious man's field jacket and cuts away his trousers. There's the sound of more gunfire not far off. It looks like the soldiers might be stuck here for a while.

With a grunt, the medic jabs his syringe into the thigh of his fallen comrade. The effect is immediate. The soldier's skin, already pale, turns gray and then white within seconds. His skin grows cold and dry. Breathing goes silent, and the pulse goes still. But the medic isn't alarmed. He knows his friend will probably be fine. He isn't dead; he's merely preserved in a safe cocoon. Call it suspended animation, slow motion, a pause button—whatever. As long as the patrol can hold off the bands of Taliban for a few more hours, there will be plenty of time to wait for the lifesaving helicopter from Bagram Air Base.

This scenario has never actually happened, but it may be closer than you think. The picture was painted for us by officials from the Defense Advanced Research Projects Agency (DARPA), a military office devoted to exploring technological breakthroughs. DARPA funds some of the most cutting-edge medical research on the planet. If you want to think of ways to truly snatch life from the jaws of death, this is a good place to start.

WHEN I ASKED DARPA officials about cheating death, I ended up in a spot that's about as far from Afghanistan as you can get, walking past luxury speedboats docked along Fairview Avenue, collar turned up against the unseasonably cold Seattle day. The city was bracing for a rare snowstorm. The Space Needle rising up behind us seemed to touch the low gray clouds, and next to it, the wild red and silver curves of the Science Fiction Museum. Turning in from the waterfront, we were on the campus of the Fred Hutchinson Cancer Research Center, five brick-and-glass buildings sitting at the base of a steep hill, tucked between the water and a concrete overpass.

On a wall of the narrow, tastefully decorated lobby sat three plaques framed in glass. These are the Nobel Prizes awarded to researchers at "the Hutch." I thought it was pretty cool, but most of the people in the lobby walked by without a glimpse. I realized this was a place where breakthroughs are expected.

I was here at the Hutch because I wanted a glimpse of what could be the biggest medical breakthrough ever—a way to stop death in its tracks. As we crowded around a glass hood in a lab room upstairs, we looked at the unwitting subject of the day's experiment: a furry white rat, all quick movements, trapped in a glass enclosure, his bright red eyes staring back at us with a hint of curiosity.

A scientist named Mark Roth also peered at the rat, his eyes squinting under a tall forehead and an unruly patch of thinning red hair. A younger colleague, Jennifer Blackwood, casual in the running clothes she wore to work, checked the gear for the experiment. Roth gave her a nod, Blackwood turned a dial, and the rat's enclosure began to fill with deadly hydrogen sulfide gas. "He has no clue," she said. The gas is invisible, but we know it's there because the rat is suddenly at attention, nose upturned and furiously sniffing at the air.

Hydrogen sulfide is the chemical that gives rotting eggs such a strong smell. An ounce could kill dozens of people.[1] At a concentration of five hundred parts per million, it's about four times as toxic as carbon monoxide,[2] but the rat doesn't seem too alarmed. For several seconds, he just keeps sniffing. On a monitor next to the enclosure, though, we can see things changing. The monitor measures the rat's output of carbon dioxide—his breathing, his metabolism. And the line is going down. Basically, Dr. Roth is turning off the rat. Not all the way, mind you—but pretty far down, like turning down the lights with a dimmer switch. Two minutes in and the rat is barely moving, just staring straight ahead. He's not quite frozen, but everything about him is going in extreme slow motion.

When Roth does this experiment for real, he can keep the rat in this state for six hours. He could probably do it even longer, but that's when he turned the experiment off. "We proved our point" is how he put it to me. We won't be around six hours later, so after about ten minutes, Blackwood turns the dial the other way, flushing the hydrogen sulfide from the rat's enclosure and replacing it with oxygen. The dimmer switch comes back up. The rat starts to move. Five minutes later, the rat is wiggling around like nothing ever happened.

Dr. Roth makes an unlikely mad scientist, with his easy smile, blue Converse sneakers, and a pullover shirt left over from his daily commute—a four-mile jog. His idea of a fun night is to sit home watching movies with his wife, teenage daughter, and ten-year-old son.[3] When the first lab mouse came back from a dose of hydrogen sulfide, Roth's first move wasn't to call DARPA or the NIH—it was rounding up everyone in the lab and going across the street for a beer. A Xeroxed picture of "the beer mouse" is still on the wall, along with oddball stickers and articles, like one about a guy who kept his wife in a freezer for six years after she died of cancer. But make no mistake: There is big stuff going on here. Maybe Nobel Prize–type stuff. It has already gotten Roth a so-called genius fellowship from the MacArthur Foundation.[4]

You see, the amazing thing isn't that you can fiddle with the dimmer switch on these lab rats and mice, it's what you can do while the lights are almost out. To come up with a pause button for death—something that would really help those soldiers in Afghanistan—you need to do some gruesome stuff. You need to mimic the wounds that a soldier might suffer from a bullet or explosion, and you have to drain the blood from your lab animals, let them die—or come close—and then find a way to put them back together. When you drain the blood from lab mice and leave them for six hours, there's no way to bring them back. When Roth did the same thing after knocking them out with hydrogen sulfide, well, it was another story. The mice were all brought back, and they all woke up. There was nothing wrong with them.

As you might imagine, the team at DARPA is pretty excited about this.[5] And so are a lot of other people. After the first experiments, Roth founded a private company, Ikaria, to turn the poison gas into medical therapies. By the time it merged with a larger company in 2007, the business was valued at $670 million.[6]

Asked what drives him, Roth chuckles. Then he says it's simple: people die, and they don't want to. "We're trying to extend survival. If you go to most physicians, they say, 'Time of death is whatever,' and you ask, 'Why did he die?' A lot of physicians will say it's because of a failure to perfuse tissues with enough oxygen. Whether it's cardiac arrest or cancer, it's the inability of blood to get to some essential organ," said Roth. "Is it true? Well, I don't know. I don't know why anyone ever dies. I think about it a lot."

Roth raises an essential question, *the* essential question: whether it's a gunshot wound or cancer, drowning or a heart attack, what do the endgames have in common? In theory, the damage from almost any injury or illness could be repaired given enough time. Massive wounds can be pieced together, and even hearts can be replaced.

It's all about time. When the heart misses a beat, an hourglass starts running. Up to now, we've been measuring time in seconds and minutes, an hour or two at most. CPR might stop the falling sand for a few *minutes*. Zeyad Barazanji and Mike Mertz are alive because someone used those precious minutes to pump on their chests, keeping blood and oxygen going to their vital organs. Anna Bagenholm got an extra three *hours*. She's alive because she was doused in a freezing stream, and her metabolism slowed enough that there was time to get her to a hospital before too many cells inside her brain and heart could die.

Seconds, minutes, hours. Sure, these are great achievements in a crisis where every second counts, but let's use our imagination to take a step further, to see if we could stop the sands of the hourglass entirely—or at least slow them to an imperceptible trickle. There are a handful of tantalizing examples, which suggest there might be a way to do just that.

One especially dramatic story of survival belongs to a thirty-five-year-old man named Mitsutaka Uchikoshi from Nishinomiya, Japan. One afternoon in October 2006, he joined colleagues from the city office for an afternoon of hiking and grilling out on Rokko mountain, part of a park near the city of Kobe. After the meal, Uchikoshi decided to walk down alone; unfortunately, he fell, struck his head on a rock, and lay undiscovered on the side of the mountain for twenty-four days. By the time he was found, he was unconscious, with an extremely faint pulse. Most of his organs weren't functioning, and his body temperature was just 71 degrees.

But within just a few hours of being taken to Kobe City General Hospital, he woke up, and a few weeks after that, Uchikoshi went home. At a press conference at the hospital, before checking out, Uchikoshi told reporters he had stayed calm throughout the whole ordeal. "On the second day, the sun was out, I was in a field, and I felt very comfortable. That's my last memory."[7] He'd been unconscious, lying in a field with no food or water, for more than three weeks. He'd survived a serious head injury, presumably from landing on a rock when he stumbled over the embankment. He'd survived massive blood loss and severe hypothermia. And in the end, he was just fine.

People like Uchikoshi teach us that the human body can

survive far more and far longer than we usually bargain for. The question is, can we harness this remarkable resilience? Can we find a way to manipulate that survival mode, to use it to our advantage, in the ER?

In the first chapters, I talked about death as a process, an ongoing chain of events that might be reversed with the right intervention. It turns out death is generally caused not directly by lack of oxygen, but by a punishing cascade of chemical reactions triggered by its absence and ultimately by its return. Lance Becker, the director of the Center for Resuscitation Science, told me, "We used to think that once the heart is restarted, our work is done. Once you're out of cardiac arrest, it's back to business as usual. But now we know that it kicks off a whole bunch of general mischief, both in the individual cells of the body and in the system as a whole."

The mischief creeps in as the minutes pass without oxygen. Cells switch to an ancient backup system: anaerobic metabolism. Chemistry buffs know it as a form of fermentation. And then something dangerous begins to happen in the mitochondria, the part of the cell that produces its energy. Becker's colleague, Dr. Ben Abella, says, "You can make an analogy to nuclear power plants. In a nuke plant, stopping production altogether is a dangerous process. So there are control rods that keep it firing at a low, controlled burn. For some reason not well understood, when we stop blood flow and deprive the mitochondria of oxygen, we start to lose the control rods."

You might be surprised to learn that it gets even worse

when oxygen is returned to the mix—for example, after a successful resuscitation. "It's a time bomb," says Abella. "When oxygen comes rushing back, the control rods are missing. It goes nuts." The resulting damage, from the addition of oxygen to the mix, is known as reperfusion injury. The reintroduction of oxygen leads to the production of a variety of toxic compounds, including free radicals and a variety of proteins, such as cytochrome c, which triggers a type of preprogrammed cell death known as apoptosis.[8]

Every cell in our body is coded with instructions for apoptosis. While it may seem counterintuitive, not to mention counterproductive, under most circumstances cell death is a beneficial, even necessary process. As we constantly grow new cells, the old ones have to go. When apoptosis malfunctions, the result is disastrous, uncontrolled growth: cancer.

Unfortunately, in the oxygen-generated chaos of reperfusion injury, apoptosis is a killer. This chain reaction—hard to stop once it gets going—has caused much frustration over the years for doctors and paramedics. They could revive patients who had been clinically dead for as long as an hour, but just getting back the heartbeat wasn't enough. The vast majority of these patients came back without meaningful brain function. They might as well have stayed dead.

What we desperately need, says Becker, is a reset button. "If you could reboot the system the way you reboot your computer, we should easily be able to save people. If we're able to achieve that it would be one of the largest revolutions in emergency care, in any kind of care, that's ever taken place."

*　　*　　*

WHEN HE WAS just getting started as a scientist, you wouldn't have pegged Mark Roth as the guy to defeat death. His father died when he was just seven years old. His mother was unable to support the family and left Roth and his six siblings to be raised in an orphanage in Hershey, Pennsylvania.[9] Life was hard but burning muscles and hungry lungs were a way out; Roth became a runner, fast enough to win a track scholarship at the University of Oregon, the hotbed of long-distance running back in the 1970s. His grades, though, weren't great. "I was exhausted from running all the time," he says. Roth managed a degree in biology, but when he took the entrance exam for medical school, his scores were so low he couldn't get in anywhere. "I didn't become a scientist out of any calling," he told me. "I had no choice."

He plugged away in fields like molecular biology, getting a few NIH grants, doing a postdoc at Johns Hopkins, but nothing that seemed to break through. It didn't bother him much, not until 1996, when something happened that changed his life.

By then Roth had moved to Seattle, and started work at the Fred Hutchinson Cancer Research Center. He and his wife were raising a young daughter, and then they had another and nothing was the same again. Hannah, the baby, had Down syndrome and a laundry list of other problems. When she was a little over a year old, she went into the hospital and never came out again.

It was only very recently that Roth has been willing to talk about the situation in public. When I asked if he thinks about his daughter every day, he told me, "It's a bit like you're driving across the country and you stop somewhere, and it's like you never left. I mean, you're still going on, but you're still there. Part of you is still there. I don't know how to put it otherwise."

Of course, I couldn't help but wonder whether it was losing a child that inspired this man to seek a way to hold back death. It's not so simple as all that, but then again, it's not so far off the mark, either. Losing Hannah sent Roth into a deep round of soul-searching, and he came to the conclusion that he'd been wasting his time. "If you don't want to lose your job, you become conservative, you keep your head down," he told me. "And it's pretty unfortunate, because without the willingness to fail, the possibility for great success is eliminated. When my daughter passed away, it occurred to me that I should play the game a little more risky. There would be a probability of failure but I shouldn't worry about that. It's okay."

Before he got into suspended animation, Roth had worked in genetics. Going way back, way before he lost a daughter, he had been interested in the science of living forever. The same way he used to take apart an alarm clock in his off-hours away from the lab, he thought about how immortality might work. "But it was like a hobby," says Roth. "It wasn't my job. My job was to do other things."

Losing Hannah gave him a sense of urgency. "I started

to study this because I wanted to make a difference in my lifetime" is how he sums it up. "Do it now" became the mantra.

And Roth told me something else that was really interesting: After all the pain, the sense of urgency felt good. It felt like freedom. "After that experience, I decided that the things that were more important to do were the things that I was actually not focused on, and I wasn't focused on them because I was pretty much afraid of failing," he says.

And so a hobby became his life's work. "I was very interested in the molecular basis of immortality. There's a small subset of cells in your body, germ cells, which have the capacity to go on to the next generation. This is the germ line—what as far as we know are immortal cells that always beget offspring as far as we know forever," said Roth. Germ cells go through a unique cycle that results in their becoming either an egg cell or sperm, depending on whether you're a man or a woman. If you successfully reproduce, an actual piece of this germ cell will live on in your offspring. It goes on forever as long as your children have their own children, and so on.

Another thing: egg cells have an interesting quality. They sit around for years without doing anything, and you can see the same phenomenon in other parts of the body. Your skin cells don't do much unless you get a cut. Then they work overtime, growing together to patch the hole. This sitting around could be viewed, in a way, as suspended animation, or quiescence, to use a favorite term of Roth's. For this next phase of his life—the making-a-difference phase—he decided to see if he could find a way to turn quiescence on and off.

Roth likes movies, and his favorite is *The Princess Bride*. There's a great scene where Westley, the hero played by Cary Elwes, is nearly tortured to death. To all appearances, he's a goner. Fortunately, his friends track down the alchemist Miracle Max, played by Billy Crystal. "It just so happens that your friend here is only *mostly* dead," Max reassures them. "There's a big difference between mostly dead and all dead. Mostly dead is slightly alive. . . ." In a scene to inspire any devotee of suspended animation, Miracle Max goes on to feed Westley the antidote, allowing him to continue in pursuit of his true love, Buttercup.

Roth says the scene comes to life in his laboratory. "The joke in my lab, when we're doing this, is 'Are they really dead?' Well, it depends—how long did you wait? Just how dead were these animals? It's kind of ridiculous, but you find yourself saying, 'That's not so dead. I can steal this piece of real estate from death.'"

When it comes to the science, the work is all about manipulating oxygen. You see, the energy-producing part of each cell is like a candle slowly burning oxygen—fuel—and turning it into water. The air we breathe is about 21 percent oxygen. At a concentration of 6 to 8 percent, death from respiratory failure will come in less than ten minutes. The same effect takes place in the blood, when oxygen levels are not replenished by breathing. That launches the chemical cascade of death in every cell.

Here is where Roth saw a loophole—a way to cheat

death: those deadly chemical reactions require the presence of *some* oxygen. Curiosity led Roth to wonder what would happen if he subtracted that oxygen from the equation. His first experiments involved fruit flies and a type of small roundworm. He gassed them with carbon monoxide, which cells take up in place of oxygen, leaving no receptors to absorb the oxygen. (This is why carbon monoxide is deadly.) The thing is, without any oxygen at all the deadly chemical reactions couldn't take place. Given a high dose of carbon monoxide, each insect froze in place, but it wasn't dead. It was like hitting the pause button on the remote. Each insect could survive twenty-four hours, then resume its business as soon as the carbon monoxide in the enclosure was replaced by oxygen.[10]

After that, Roth turned his attention to the zebrafish. Zebrafish, like fruit flies and roundworms, are considered "model animals," which means their biology and development are extremely well understood. Scientists study embryonic development in zebrafish because they develop from eggs into tiny fish larvae in just three days. The fish also develop outside the mother, making them easy to work with. Roth put a zebrafish embryo in a sealed bag, along with a chemical that essentially sucked all the oxygen out of the embryo's body and converted it into water. Without oxygen, the embryo stopped growing. Its heart stopped beating, but it didn't "die." When Roth restored the oxygen a day later, the embryo picked up where it had left off. By day four—instead of day three—it was a baby zebrafish, indistinguishable from any other.[11]

Says Roth, "When you reduce oxygen levels to a certain point, you kill [the organism]. But when you reduce it one hundredfold *past* the point that kills them, they do fine." When carbon monoxide took the place of oxygen in each cell, the damaging chemical reactions simply couldn't take place. It made me think of smothering a fire—burning being another chemical reaction that requires oxygen.

It was the same with roundworms. With an intermediate oxygen concentration—what Roth calls "evil oxygen tension"—they would suffer a version of reperfusion injury and die. But in an atmosphere of 0.1 percent oxygen, "there's a state of suspended animation. And if you put them back into room air, they resume all their life processes as if it never happened," said Roth.

It was weird stuff. Stuff that seemed like it might fit better in the Science Fiction Museum, the roof of which is visible from the back window of Roth's lab. Even now, he shakes his head with amazement: "We wait a week without doing anything, and then they just start going again. And we're just... wow!"

What does it mean to hit the pause button like that? "It sort of starts to get philosophical," he says. "As far as we know, if you were this creature, you'd be here, and then you'd be here, and somebody would say, 'You know, it's no longer Sunday. It's Tuesday, Bob.' And you'd be like, 'I don't know that. For me, it's just Sunday.' "

After the worms and the flies and the zebrafish, Roth was ready to move up to mammals, but first he made a few changes. Inspired by a documentary about Mexican caves that contain hydrogen sulfide gas, Roth decided to use that compound in place of carbon monoxide.[12] Hydrogen sulfide has a near-identical action in the body and is equally deadly, but it clings less tightly to the body's red blood cells. That makes it easier to reverse the suspended animation effect when the time is right. (For the same reason, it is easier to reverse a potentially deadly case of hydrogen sulfide poisoning than a case of carbon monoxide poisoning.)[13]

Roth had reason to think it would work. People who spend time around hydrogen sulfide—workers in paper mills, for example, or people who explore caves—occasionally suffer what's known as a knockdown. They get a whiff of the gas, and *boom,* they're out. If they're alone, it's bad news. If someone happens to be nearby and sees the knockdown, and help arrives to pull the victim into fresh air—well, they snap out of it. No memory, but no problem.[14]

With the worms and the fish, it was real suspended animation. Roth had turned off the lights. With the mice, he would turn the dimmer down, but not all the way. There would still be a faint glow, sort of like turning off the stove but leaving the pilot light on to burn.

In Roth's lab, when he turned the dial, the hydrogen sulfide produced an immediate effect. The first mouse to get it saw its metabolism drop by half in just five minutes. Within six hours, it was about 10 percent of normal. The mouse was taking ten breaths per minute, rather than the normal 120. Its body temperature fell from 37 degrees Celsius (the same as a person) to just 15 degrees Celsius. Four hours after room air was reintroduced, the mouse was back to normal.[15]

The work in Roth's laboratory had caught the attention of DARPA, which was looking for ways to ramp up medical capability on the new battlefields of central Asia. The Surviving Blood Loss Program was near the top of the wish list. Blood loss has been the leading cause of death in war, since at least the Civil War. Mostly thanks to improvements in response time and field hospitals, the proportion of troops who survive their wounds is higher, by far, in Iraq and Afghanistan than in any previous conflict the world has ever seen.[16] But blood loss still takes its toll. Not only is it responsible for the majority of deaths, but many of the survivors also face severe brain injuries due to lack of oxygen from blood loss.

When it comes to helping soldiers, there are special constraints. Any tool has to be simple and small enough to carry in a medic's pack. Jon Mogford, program director for the Surviving Blood Loss Program, says the military was looking for a silver bullet, something that could be administered in a single syringe. "Imagine that no help is on the way, fluids are gone and running low—we want to give [the medic] another tool to help save that soldier and buy time." Buying time, that's the goal. "Imagine being in the mountains of Afghanistan and compare that to a typical EMS pickup in the United States," said Mogford.

Even under the wing of the military, DARPA faces the same rules as academic or private research. Medics can't start packing a new drug unless it has the same FDA approval as any other new medication.[17] That means starting in animal models. In Phase 1 of the Surviving Blood Loss Program, researchers would have to drain 60 percent of a rat's blood in forty minutes and leave the rat for six hours before attempting resuscitation. With no medical intervention, the death rate is 100 percent. To pass Phase 1, a research team would have to bring the survival rate to 75 percent. The time frame: two years. The Roth lab did it.[18]

Since that early success Ikaria has taken important steps towards making hydrogen sulfide a usable medication. After mice there were experiments in dogs and pigs, which found that hydrogen sulfide reduced the damage from simulated heart attacks.[19] It's done a bit differently in large animals—instead of a gas, they're given a solution of sodium sulfide which breaks down to hydrogen sulfide almost immediately after entering the bloodstream. And the effect is not nearly so dramatic—this is *not* suspended animation. But the promise is still tremendous.

Most exciting, while I struggle to wrap my mind around this, hydrogen sulfide has already been tested in human subjects. These early clinical trials, strictly to test safety and determine the proper dosage, found no significant harmful effects.[20] As *Cheating Death* is being written, the next round of human trials is just being launched—using hydrogen sulfide as an experimental treatment for heart attack and acute kidney injury.[21]

Dr. David Lefer at Emory University, who has worked with hydrogen sulfide and done work that's similar to

Roth's, says he was surprised—and disappointed—to learn that it was so difficult to put animals larger than mice into suspended animation.[22] He speculates that swine—or people—may process the drug differently. He says suspended animation may someday be an option, but it will probably take a combination of drugs, and vastly more research. Still, he's excited about the possibilities. In his own studies, mice given hydrogen sulfide suffered far less damage from simulated heart attacks.[23] Intriguingly, even if they were given a miniscule dose—so small it was undetectable within 15 seconds—the protective effect was still there, 24 hours later.[24] If the same effect were seen in humans, it could be a major help for transplant surgeons, who could give patients a dose of hydrogen sulfide a day before performing extensive, risky surgery.

Whether the goal is suspended animation or a more mundane version, the principle is the same. When the body isn't getting enough oxygen, you lower the need for oxygen—with poison gas, that's the weird part. Hearing Roth explain this is more like watching a science fiction movie than reading a medical journal. "What you want to do is have the patient's time slow down, while everyone around them moves at what we would call real time," he said.

Suspended animation has the ring of science fiction, but the basic concept is not so exotic. Think about hibernation. Bears famously spend the winter months more or less in slumber. But hibernation is common to a huge range of animal species, from frogs to turtles to certain birds like the bar-headed goose to mammals including squirrels, bears, and hedgehogs. In times when food is scarce and energy needs—keeping warm—are greater, these animals go into survival mode. Some of the adaptations go beyond simple hibernation; one type of squirrel, the Arctic ground squirrel, produces a chemical that allows its body temperature to drop below freezing without ill effects.[25]

Typically, hibernation is linked to two things: cold or body fat. Survival mode is triggered either when body temperature drops below a certain level or when the animal has packed on enough extra calories to last it through the winter. For this reason, hibernation times can vary. A bear will keep eating until it's fat enough to survive the winter. During a winter that's relatively warm, some ground squirrels won't hibernate at all. Make it a cold one and they might snooze from November to March.

In general, hibernation is a state where the need for energy is radically reduced. In ground squirrels, metabolism drops to about 1 percent of normal levels. A squirrel running up trees (or through your attic) and gathering nuts for winter burns as much oxygen and calories in fifteen minutes as a hibernating squirrel burns all day and night. Not only is this fascinating science, but think about what it could mean for human survival. In a case of cardiac arrest, heart and brain tissue die because the lack of oxygen triggers a calamitous chemical chain reaction within our cells. If our body's need for oxygen was 1/1000 of what it is, the process would unfold in super–slow motion. That damaging chain reaction might barely have time to get started by the time we reach a hospital and doctors shock us back to life.

Until recently, it was thought that primates—monkeys, apes, and also humans—weren't capable of such a dramatic transformation. But in 2004, animal physiologists in Marburg, Germany, revealed evidence of hibernation among dwarf lemurs living on the island of Madagascar off Africa. In the journal *Nature*, they wrote that these small primates spend several months a year dozing in tree holes, their body temperature drifting with the air temperature outside.[26] Now, here is something to consider: this state of hibernation isn't triggered by freezing cold. In fact, Madagascar has a pretty inviting year-round climate; it rarely gets colder than about 50 degrees Fahrenheit.

These languid lemurs may be smaller and furrier than we are, but in the family of nature, the lemur is a pretty close relative of human beings. The Marburg finding suggests the intriguing idea that other primates, including humans, might have instructions for hibernation somehow coded into our genes. In fact, it turns out we do have a lot in common not only with monkeys, but also other animals, including ground squirrels.

Dr. Matt Andrews heads the Department of Biology at the University of Minnesota in Duluth, where he spends a lot of time thinking about ground squirrels. October is his favorite time of year, watching squirrels get fat for winter and dropping off to hibernate one by one. Andrews has a mischievous grin and an offbeat sense of humor. In our first five minutes on the phone, I learned that Goldy Gopher—mascot of the UMN sports teams—actually has the exact physical characteristics of a thirteen-lined ground squirrel and that Lawrence Welk bought his first accordion by saving up bounty money, a dollar at a time, from hunting ground squirrels and turning their skins in to state hunting officials. Ground squirrels used to be considered quite a pest in Minnesota—they still are by many people—but they've also become the focus of some heavy-duty research.

Andrews, along with two UMN colleagues, is an adviser to a company called VitalMedix, which has gotten financial support from DARPA (the same military agency that funded the early suspended animation experiments of Mark Roth) and is currently working with the Army and Navy drug development offices.[27] VitalMedix is looking to develop a way to trigger hibernation in humans. Squirrels are the perfect research subject: they're easy to find, you can keep them anywhere and they'll eat anything. The Minnesota group feeds their squirrels pet food, Purina rat chow. They're also easy to work with, at least compared to some research subjects. "We don't do bears, because then you might have an experimental subject that would eat you," says Andrews.

The study of hibernation in a way completes a circle for Andrews. As a graduate student at Central Michigan University in the late 1970s, he got his start by studying how the heart could function at low body temperatures. As part of that research, he got interested in molecular biology, especially how genes effectively turn on and off.

The genetic basis of hibernation was laid out in a 1998 paper, which identified genes that were triggered by a certain level of fat in the squirrel's body. Since then, says

Andrews, "We haven't found a single gene in the ground squirrel sequence that isn't in a person."

Having the genes isn't the whole story, of course. Otherwise we'd all pack it in after Thanksgiving dinner and wake up around Easter. As we've seen in many fields of science and medicine, just as important as the genetic sequence are the triggers that "turn on" the relevant genes. The Minnesota team also knew that it would be unrealistic to instigate gene therapy on someone who just crashed their car or was bleeding out on the battlefield. They would need a shortcut. They would have to identify the molecular substances that actually carry out the body's order to enter survival mode.

"In 2002, DARPA contacted us about taking this approach to come up with ways to help the wounded soldier," explains Andrews. "If a soldier suffers profound blood loss, we'd come up with a cocktail of ingredients that would essentially buy time for the injured soldier—more than just the minutes that CPR could buy or even the hours provided by hypothermia. DARPA was looking for more time than ever before, for the injured from an improvised explosive device (IED) explosion in Afghanistan to the car accident victim in Minnesota." In essence, they were looking for near-instant hibernation.

What VitalMedix came up with is a drug called Tamiasyn. It includes two vital components: an antioxidant to try and slow the damaging chain reaction that occurs when oxygen is removed from cells and an alternate energy source for these oxygen-deprived cells, so they won't die. Finding the alternative fuel was an especially tough challenge, but Andrews found an interesting answer. He had noticed hibernating animals have high levels of ketone bodies, which are by-products that naturally occur when the body breaks down fatty acids during digestion. During hibernation, when digestion is unfolding in super–slow motion or not taking place at all, ketone bodies provide an additional source of fuel.[28] All of a sudden, suspended animation doesn't sound like a science fiction novel. It is more like a biochemistry textbook.

Another adviser to VitalMedix is Dr. Greg Beilman, a professor of surgery at the University of Minnesota and a colonel in the Army Reserves. He's performed dozens of surgeries on battle-injured soldiers in Iraq and Kosovo. "My interest is personal," he said. "I got interested in this after my deployment to Kosovo in 2000. There were a couple of things we worked on there: better ways to resuscitate people in the field and also how to better use resources in a field situation. I mean, when you're in Afghanistan, six hours from a combat hospital, what's the best way to stop the bleeding?"

You can't hike around an Afghan mountain range with a cooling box and a supply of chilled saline. You need something the medic can deploy when it's pitch black and someone is shooting at his head—a drug that can be administered quickly and easily. In experiments on rats and pigs, Tamiasyn shows promise. The animals got the drug after going into shock from blood loss but before there was any attempt at resuscitation. In both kinds of animals, it lengthened survival time, and organ function actually improved as opposed to getting worse.

Suspended animation and hibernation are two experimental approaches to saving trauma victims, but there are others, including the use of female hormones. It sounds pretty strange, but I was actually the coauthor on one of these studies, with colleagues at Grady Memorial Hospital in Atlanta. We found that giving the hormone progesterone led to better recoveries for people who suffer head injuries. Research on animals goes further; with the help of funding from DARPA, Dr. Irshad Chaudry at the University of Alabama at Birmingham has found that small doses of the female hormone progesterone can sharply improve survival from everything from sepsis to blood loss to cardiac arrest.[29]

Some doctors believe that progesterone evolved to function as a protection against blood loss in mammals, which often lose large amounts of blood during childbirth.[30] Jon Mogford of DARPA says the action of progesterone is actually more complicated than hydrogen sulfide. "Probably it's a combination of anti-inflammatory mechanisms, preventing cell death and also controlling blood flow. We don't know how it's doing that in hemorrhagic shock, but it's valid to presume that it would help survival."

Yet another approach involves—you might have guessed it—extreme hypothermia. A surgeon named Hasan Alam, at Massachusetts General Hospital, let us watch one of the surgeries. The test subjects are pigs. Alam knocks them out

with an anesthetic, opens the chest, slices open the aorta—
sometimes other major organs, too—and quickly drains
about 60 percent of the pig's blood. After a wait of thirty
minutes, he inserts a catheter directly to the aorta and
starts a pump that fills the animal's heart and blood supply
with a chilled solution of organ preservation fluid: a mixture of electrolytes and antioxidants that are typically used
to extend the life of organs used in transplant operations.
Forget moderation; Alam brings the temperature down
to about 10 degrees Celsius (or 50 degrees Fahrenheit). It
takes almost an hour to get the pigs that cold.

At that point, he gets to the real work. "I can stop the
[heart] pump. They have almost no blood in the body, no
brain activity, no heartbeat, and it gives me plenty of time
to fix the underlying injuries," said Alam. Under normal
circumstances, the internal injuries and massive blood loss
would invariably be fatal to pigs, or to humans, for that
matter, but in Alam's lab, every single test pig has survived.
A few days after surgery, he puts each pig through a few
paces to assess their cognitive functioning. As best as he
can tell, they suffer no brain damage at all. Even under the
microscope, the brain cells show no sign of damage.[31]

If it works in people, this sort of procedure could
have a huge impact in a hospital emergency room. Trauma
is the leading cause of death for people under fifty and kills
more under thirty-five than all other causes combined.[32]
Alam said, "If somebody comes in tonight after getting shot
in the chest, I'll open the chest to control bleeding. If I can
control it in just a few minutes, I think they'll live. If it's

more like five minutes, they'll probably die. But if I can get the brain temperature down like this, I'll have more like two hours."

What all these approaches have in common is that they tinker with the cellular machinery that processes oxygen. Think back to what Lance Becker teaches: in a medical crisis like traumatic blood loss or cardiac arrest, it's not just the loss of oxygen, but the body's reaction that's dangerous. Estrogen minimizes this reaction. Hypothermia puts it into slow motion. Hydrogen sulfide perhaps can stop the reaction altogether.

If it all sounds far-fetched, especially the approach using hydrogen sulfide, remember that nature is full of creatures that can turn off the need to breathe. They're everywhere. You can even find an example on the back of a comic book, next to the ads for X-ray specs and action figures. I'm talking about the mail-order ads for creatures called Sea-Monkeys. They're actually a tiny kind of shrimp, marketed as "instant life" or "real live fun pets you grow yourself." Sea-Monkeys can survive without oxygen, in cysts, for as long as four years. Drop them into water, and as the sales pitch says, you get instant life for about three dollars, plus shipping and handling.

It may be that creatures like this provide real clues to solving the puzzle of suspended animation. One person who believes this is Dr. Philip Bickler, an anesthesiologist at the University of California, San Francisco, Medical Center. In the operating room, he monitors patients during high-risk surgeries to repair brain aneurysms. An aneurysm is a blister on a blood vessel in the brain, caused by a weakening of the blood vessel wall. Sometimes, to fix it, a neurosurgeon has to first stop blood from flowing to the spot, usually by using a simple clip on the vessel.

Since this cuts off blood flow to the affected part of the brain, the procedure carries the risk of brain damage. The same thing happens if the heart fails. "It's usually said that if the heart stops beating, you'll have severe neurological damage if it lasts more than five minutes," says Bickler. "We try to buy more time." To buy time, the anesthesiologist will try to reduce the brain's need for oxygen with a mix of powerful drugs. Unfortunately, this safeguard doesn't always work. During high-risk brain surgeries, a significant number of patients emerge with brain damage due to lack of oxygen.[33]

During a small number of extremely complex surgeries lasting an hour or more, some patients are put into deep hypothermia, much like Hasan Alam did in his swine experiments. For more routine aneurysm repairs, a number of doctors have tried the more modest version of hypothermia, cooling the brain to 33 degrees Celsius, but surprisingly—to Bickler, at least—a large clinical trial on this found no benefit.

Like many doctors, Bickler had put a lot of faith in hypothermia. He decided to try and piece together what went wrong. When he thought about the experiment and why it failed, he reasoned that it must be because the bulk of the brain damage wasn't taking place *while* the oxygen was cut off, which is when the patients were being cooled. The damage was coming *afterward,* caused by the body's reaction to oxygen deprivation. Bickler figured that the same thing must be happening in people who suffered cardiac arrest.

Bickler's particular interest is blood chemistry, and his focus was on how that chemistry changes after the body is deprived of oxygen. We've seen that even a few minutes without oxygen will trigger a devastating cycle of inflammation and cell death, but it's not exactly clear *why* that is so. Some lab rats, for example, can go without oxygen much longer than humans can before suffering brain damage.[34]

Many reptiles are even more resistant. Bickler's current research looks at painted turtles, the kind you find in a pet store. Turtles breathe air, but in the wild during the winter, painted turtles will often burrow in the mud, without breathing for as long as four months. Low temperature is part of it, says Bickler, but not all. "Even when they're warm, their tolerance of oxygen deprivation is about ten thousand times what it is in humans. The neurons in their brain are capable of entering a state of suspended animation when oxygen is not available. It's essentially a reflex," said Bickler. "If you force him [a turtle] to dive underwater, he'll stay active for a number of hours, but then he'll enter a state of quiescence, where he's just minimally responsive. The metabolism is reduced to what I'd call a pilot-light level. It's about one-tenth of 1 percent of normal."

The turtles stay in this state all winter, about four months. After just a few hours, Bickler has found, the animal has actually consumed every bit of oxygen in its tissues. It's surviving on no oxygen at all. What we don't know is just how it works. Bickler thinks the secret lies somewhere in the chemistry of calcium and potassium, which drive the basic energy production in each cell.

Bickler has an unusual background for a physician; he started off as a marine biologist. At the world-famous Scripps Institution of Oceanography in San Diego, he marveled at the adaptations various animals made to survive. When we first spoke, he told me about a creature called the Antarctic ice fish. It lives along the sandy sea bottom, underneath the ice shelves of Antarctica, in temperatures which dip below 30 degrees Fahrenheit (the ocean's salt content keeps it from freezing at 32 degrees Fahrenheit). To manage this trick, the fish actually produces a type of antifreeze in its blood, which prevents ice crystals from forming. It also manages to circulate oxygen without using red blood cells; this makes the blood more fluid and conserves energy in the extremely harsh conditions. Asked if we might artificially produce the same effect in people, Bickler points to isoflurane, a common anesthesia drug. It's used in surgeries where the patient is cooled, because it seems to protect cells at low temperatures—by affecting the balance of potassium, if you are wondering.

Bickler says, "I've been an anesthesiologist for twenty years, but my heart is still with those turtles and fish and hibernating creatures." They're still a part of his professional life; in 2008, he won a grant for a study of diving marine mammals—whales and dolphins—to examine how their neurons can adapt to low oxygen levels. Some marine mammals will stay underwater for more than an hour while hunting for food.

Bickler switched to the study of medicine to see if he could find a practical application for some of this biology. If animals could survive harsh conditions by lowering their body temperature or slowing their metabolism, perhaps there was a way for humans to trigger the same survival mechanisms in their own bodies. Bickler is an avid mountain climber, and had already seen the human body is more adaptable than many people know. In air as thin as it is on top of Mount Everest, an unacclimated climber would be dead in an hour. But it's a different story for expert climbers who train for months before an ascent and work their way up the mountain by staying for a few days at each successive altitude. These mountaineers manage not only to survive, but to survive without the help of supplemental oxygen, even while climbing to the summit of Mount Everest.[35] What Bickler eventually hopes to find is a way to speed up those adaptations in a way that might be utilized as part of emergency medical care. Perhaps we can develop a drug that's akin to the chemicals naturally found in a turtle, which would give us some of that same amazing survival ability.

In his lab in Philadelphia, Lance Becker is thinking something similar. He says that all the death pathways, all the mischief, all the chemical chaos, seems to take place in the mitochondria—the part of the cell that produces energy. Some evolutionary biologists say death, the way we know it, didn't even exist until cells became complex enough to include mitochondria. These scientists say the mitochondria in our cells actually evolved from primitive bacteria. Bacteria do not have mitochondria and do not undergo apoptosis. They simply divide, again and again, as long as conditions are favorable. Bacteria might be eaten or destroyed, but otherwise, they just hang around, becoming spores or entering some other form of quiescence.

Becker's focus is on clinical practice—how to stop or reverse the death pathways when the body is deprived of oxygen due to cardiac arrest, trauma, or some other cause. Hypothermia is one tool, so is CPR. The next step, he says, could be drugs like the ones being tested in Mark Roth's laboratory. Hydrogen sulfide does work on the mitochondria, binding itself to the electrons within that organism. Says Becker, "A number of us are pursuing this very similar science."

When we spoke, Roth contrasted his approach to what EMTs typically do when they arrive to help a cardiac arrest victim. "The very first thing they do is to slap a mask on their face and give them 100 percent oxygen. But perhaps another idea could be tried," he says. "That is to take away the little bit of rope they're using to hang themselves, to prevent them from using the little bit of oxygen that's killing them."

When Roth looks around this world, he sees hints of immortality everywhere: in hibernating squirrels, in skiers who survive a plunge through the ice, in the spores of bacteria, in the seeds of plants and in our own bodies. He sees immortality as inextricably linked with quiescence.

Quiescence, as he describes it, is a state of unchanging readiness. Again he says, "Look at female germ cells [eggs] in an ovary, all sitting there like a fireman waiting to fight fires. Only one a month, of a bazillion, goes out. The others sit in the fire station, doing nothing, for decades at a time."

In smaller and simpler organisms, we find examples so stark that they fall in a different category. Some bacteria spores—including dangerous ones, like anthrax—can last for years without any outside nourishment in a complete unchanging state. Many viruses do the same. Eggs, seeds, spores, viruses—what these hold is the *potential* for life. Says Roth, "All these things with proliferation potential seem to have this remarkable quality, which is that they can sit in suspended animation for this remarkable period of time."

One thing to keep in mind—as a treatment for humans or other mammals, hydrogen sulfide as used by Ikaria does not induce suspended animation, the way it does in roundworms. It's still the dimmer switch. For now, Roth says he just wants to develop a drug that can be used in a conventional medical setting, alongside other therapies like hypothermia. But I couldn't help but wonder: is it really impossible to think that we might someday stop time—put humans into suspended animation, the way Roth did with his baby zebrafish?

"Of course that [research] is far more in its infancy," says Roth. "For now I think it's more straightforward to enable the physician to utilize this technology by simply dimming the patient, rather than starting from an extreme

situation where they lose a lot of control that they have."
But with a mischievous grin, Roth admits he doesn't really
know how far this could go.

" 'Clinical death' might be the loss of a heartbeat, and
with those fish, I turn off the heartbeat so they *are* clinically dead. But I can bring them back. So they must not
have been dead," he chuckles. To even try this in humans,
to push suspended animation to its limits, would require a
wholesale change in how we view the practice of medicine.
Imagine a patient with no heartbeat, no blood pressure, no
vital signs. Is she dead? Who can say? What doctor would
try that experiment?

"You have to think about separating the connection
between life and animation, between death and deanima-
tion," says Roth. "We've put them together, but I think from
these research studies, those are not reasonable connections to be drawing. Not always."

Roth's company Ikaria takes its name from an ancient
Greek island renowned for its ancient, medicinal sulfur
springs. The philosopher Herodotus was an early advocate,
as was his pupil Hippocrates, the father of modern medicine. It's not a stretch to say that Roth enjoys tempting fate.
The island Ikaria takes its name from the famed Icarus of
Greek mythology. Icarus flew on giant wings built by his
father, the master craftsman Daedalus. Ignoring a warning
not to soar too high, Icarus sailed toward the sun, only for
its heat to melt the wax that held together his wings, which
sent him plunging to his death in the sea below.

Mark Roth isn't afraid to soar, but when he decided to

"do it now," his goals were pretty simple: Make a difference. Save lives. In his typically low-key way of talking, he told me, "If I was able to do something that helped someone out during a difficult moment, that would be good. I would be happy with that." If it took starting a company to make it happen, well then, so be it. "It wasn't going to be enough for me to just publish a paper suggesting the possibility. I wanted to actually do it."

What we've seen, here in Seattle, may be the key to the whole puzzle—a way to dim the lights, slow the candle, stop time, cheat death. "I think the whole of emergency medicine is a time-dependent thing," says Roth. "Someone either has time or they don't. Ask a doctor, and it's always a question of 'I could have done this, if only I had the time to do it. If only I could have gotten him in the OR, and done this, and that.'" He's getting pretty worked up, gesturing with his hands. "Can we fix *anything*? That might be going too far. But things that can't be fixed now, we could fix with more time. There's no question."

CHAPTER FOUR

Beyond Death

The silver cord was not for ever loosed, nor the golden bowl irreparably broken. But where, meantime, was the soul?

—Edgar Allan Poe, "The Premature Burial"

THE SPARKLING SUMMER day was in sharp contrast to Duane Dupre's mood as he trimmed back pine tree limbs in the backyard of his trim bungalow.[1] Dupre was forty years old with an eighteen-year-old daughter and a twelve-year-old son. Having a girl going off to college was stressful enough and so was managing three grocery stores. Doing yard work was usually a release. Today, it wasn't. Texas-born and Texas-bred, Dupre was used to the heat, but this day he was feeling every ounce of the 240 pounds that he carried on his not quite six-foot frame. Sweat held his shirt to his chest and across his shoulders, and he could feel pangs of heartburn, or indigestion, shooting through his midsection. Once or twice he'd stopped to rest, but that just made the pain sharper. Oh well, he thought, better to work and distract myself.

Heaving a sigh, Dupre folded his ladder, packed his clippers, and moved on to the swimming pool. After just a few minutes of sweeping the bottom, he decided to call it a day. Damn, it was hot! Wiping his forehead, Dupre headed inside. The indigestion was really starting to burn, so over a cold glass of water, Dupre picked up the phone and called his doctor to ask if there was something he might do for the pain. He'd had a prescription before, no big deal. But when his doctor called back, it brought another headache— telling him to go to the emergency room. Just a precaution, mind you.

He wouldn't have gone, but it was too damn hot to do anything else. Dupre drove himself in ten minutes to the hospital and told his story at the desk. That's when things started to move a bit faster. A concerned-looking nurse took him by the arm, ahead of the people waiting, through the door and down a dim hallway. Five minutes later, in an exam room, a young doctor was telling Dupre that there might be something happening with his heart. To make sure everything was okay, he ought to have an angiogram.

"How about Wednesday?" asked Dupre.

The doctor smiled for some reason and said that Wednesday wouldn't do. "You need to understand something, Mr. Dupre. You may be having a heart attack."

Dupre was dubious, but his chest was really hurting. On a hospital phone, he called his sister, who happened to be the head nurse in the hospital's cardiac unit. She sounded worried and told her brother to get moving.

At least it was cool in the hospital, but Dupre could still

feel sweat as he wiped his brow. Two cardiologists came in and started filling out forms. By that point, Dupre was rattled. He knew he had a belly, didn't exercise much, and could stand to eat a whole lot better, but was he really having a heart attack? His esophagus was on fire; the flames were shooting right up his gullet now. To try and ease the pain, he recalls, "I leaned back on the gurney. And I was gone."

Now, the medical records tell a pretty clear story of what happened next. For the next twenty-eight minutes, Duane Dupre was in a fight for his life. He'd been felled by a massive heart attack, a 100 percent blockage in his right ventricle. Only a trickle of blood pumped through his veins, and a team of nurses and cardiologists went through every trick in the book to get it moving again. They started CPR straight away, pressing down so hard that they cracked three of Dupre's ribs. They grabbed defibrillator pads and shocked him six times in those twenty-eight minutes until a heartbeat meekly returned.

At that point, the team threw Dupre on a stretcher, wheeled him to the cath lab, and did an angioplasty. The doctor threaded a tiny balloon through an incision and snaked it through the blood vessels to Dupre's heart, where he slowly inflated the balloon to open the dam of plaque that blocked the artery. The trickle turned into a normal flow, and pink returned to the patient's cheeks. "They saved my life," Dupre says now. He was able to relay that story with such stunning detail that I felt like I had gotten a real glimpse of that fine line between life and death.

But that wasn't all. Dupre told me there was in fact more to the story. In his telling, something happened in those twenty-eight minutes that the doctors and nurses and medical technicians in the room weren't even faintly aware of. As the ribs were cracking, as the frantic medical team called out marching orders, Dupre felt himself watching from a perch a few feet above them, surrounded by a warm and blissful feeling.

Dupre struggles for the words to explain what it was like. "It's complicated, but it was the calmest, the most peaceful, the most relaxing, the most safe place I've ever been." While the doctors struggled over his body, the medical bay slipped away. Dupre found himself in a huge, old-fashioned waiting room full of wooden tables and chairs. "Have you ever seen the old black-and-white pictures of Ellis Island? Big, massive windows, high up, with lots of light coming in?" Like the Great Hall at Ellis Island, there were rows and rows of old tables, but there was also a row of lamps hanging from long cords. The lights were off, except for a single lamp about three-quarters of the way through the room.

"I was the only person there. I was dressed for work. I knew exactly what I was doing there, so I sat and waited," said Dupre. "I wasn't scared or apprehensive. It was a very natural place to be. I kept sitting, even though my name was called two or three times. And then I woke up, and there were people running down the hall, sitting on my chest, banging on me."

What Dupre went through is usually called a near-death experience, or NDE. If death is a tenuous line in the sand,

NDEers are people who seemingly were swept away by the tide—only to emerge alive from the pounding surf. Going by the published research it seems that anywhere from 10 to 20 percent of Americans say they've had a near-death experience. Casual surveys put the number much higher.

I first heard the term near-death experience in the 1990s, during my neurosurgery training at the university hospital in Ann Arbor, Michigan, but the term long predates that. It was originally coined by Dr. Raymond Moody in his best-selling 1975 exploration *Life After Life*. Moody became interested in the topic while he was an undergraduate philosophy student at the University of Virginia. In an interview he said he first heard of NDEs from the psychiatrist George Ritchie, who had a near-death experience when suffering severe pneumonia as an army private during World War II.[2] Moody soon met several other people who told him about their near-death experiences. For example, a patient who suffered cardiac arrest said that as doctors and nurses were pounding on his chest, he tried to tell them, "Leave me alone. All I want is to be left alone.... I tried to move their hands to keep them from beating on my body, but nothing would happen. I couldn't get anywhere. It was like—I don't really know what happened, but I couldn't move their hands. It looked like I was touching their hands and I tried to move them."

Moody, who wrote his best seller while still a medical student at the University of Georgia, identified several consistent characteristics in the stories people told about what happened when they died.[3] Not every experience includes each one of the signature traits, but Moody noticed several common features. The first signal of death, he wrote, is usually a loud, unpleasant noise:

> A man is dying and, as he reaches the point of greatest physical distress, he hears himself pronounced dead by his doctor. He begins to hear an uncomfortable noise, a loud ringing or buzzing, and at the same time feels himself moving very rapidly through a long, dark tunnel. After this, he suddenly finds himself outside of his own physical body, but still in the immediate physical environment, and he sees his own body from a distance, as though he is a spectator. He watches the resuscitation attempt from this unusual vantage point and is in a state of emotional upheaval.
>
> After a while, he collects himself and becomes more accustomed to his odd condition. He notices that he still has a "body," but one of a very different nature and with very different powers from the physical body he has left behind. Soon other things begin to happen. Others come to meet and to help him. He glimpses the spirits of relatives and friends who have already died, and a warm, loving spirit of a kind he has encountered before—a being of light—appears before him. This being asks him a question, nonverbally, to make him evaluate his life and helps him along by showing him a panoramic, instantaneous playback of the major events of his life. At

some point he finds himself approaching some kind of barrier or border, apparently representing the limit between earthly life and the next life. Yet, he finds that he must go back to the earth, that the time for his death had not yet come. At this point he resists, by now he is taken up with his experiences in the afterlife and does not want to return. He is overwhelmed by intense feelings of joy, love and peace. Despite his attitude, though, he somehow reunites with his physical body and lives.

As A DOCTOR, it is somewhat chilling to hear this described so vividly, but the notion of a soul as separate from the body is as ancient as humankind, part and parcel of nearly every religion, from the *Tibetan Book of the Dead* to the ancient Hindu Upanishads to the prophet Isaiah in the Old Testament: "Thy dead men shall live, together with my dead body shall they arise" (Isaiah 26:19).

In *Phaedo,* Plato weighs whether "the body comes to be separated by itself apart from the soul, and the soul comes to be separated from itself" or if the soul simply dissolves. In *The Republic*, he recounts the near-death experience of Er, a soldier, who is apparently slain on the battlefield but later makes a return.

For all the mentions in religion and philosophy, it's Moody's description of life after death that holds sway. The near-death experience, as he describes it, is deeply embedded in our popular culture—from new age books about angels to sophisticated films like *All That Jazz.* Who can forget the climactic song-and-dance number? Choreographer and director Bob Fosse made this autobiographical film about his own hard-driving life and near-fatal heart attack. In the film, Fosse's alter ego, played by Roy Scheider, does not make it out of the hospital, but before he dies he gets the full near-death treatment—a soft-voiced, white-robed woman; a long white tunnel (looking much like an MRI machine); even a full "life review" in the form of stage patter by Ben Vereen ("A so-so entertainer. Not much of a humanitarian. And this cat wasn't never nobody's friend")...and Vereen's thrilling song-and dance-number, "Bye, Bye Life."

TO BE SURE, most people who "die," who suffer cardiac arrest even for a few minutes, do not remember anything at all of the experience. For Zeyad Barazanji, there's a completely blank space from the moment he stepped off the treadmill until he woke up in the hospital two weeks later. And yet, whether it's the one in six from controlled studies or the 42 percent of adults in one physician's widely read survey, millions of Americans have experienced NDEs. What happened to them?

I always thought that the answer would come from the realm of religion or philosophy, so I was a little surprised to meet people who are confident that science, traditional medical science, can explain the phenomenon. We were introduced to Duane Dupre by one of these scientists, an emergency physician named Sam Parnia, whose research passion is the study of near-death experience. You might picture someone whose office is full of crystals or who lives in a yurt, but we found Parnia roaming the halls of New York-Presbyterian Hospital/Weill Cornell Medical Center, one of the premier centers of academic medicine in the country.

"What is death? What do we experience? Ultimately, whether we like it or not, all of us will be confronted with this eventually." Parnia went on, bursting with boyish enthusiasm. "What is it likely to be for us? Maybe some old-school types say it should be left to philosophy. I disagree. I say everything should be studied by science."

An emergency physician by training, Parnia grew interested in death while he was still a medical student in Southampton, England. "For some reason, I became fascinated with the whole mind-body problem. What makes me, me? You, you? What makes the self?" As he watched newborn babies enter the world, Parnia became interested in the question of when consciousness begins and how thought arises from brain cells. As a young medical student on other hospital rotations, he found himself confronted with death on a regular basis for the first time.[4]

"I started to see people die in front of me," Parnia said. "Hospitals were very used to the idea, but I was very much affected by the fact that we would make decisions about how to proceed, how aggressive to be [with dying patients]—without any real science about what death meant or any input from these people."

I think most doctors don't take enough time to reflect on death. No doubt, as members of a profession dedicated to preserving life, death can be viewed simply as a failure, not doing the job we hoped we could. It is more than that, though. Anytime I see a patient die, I'm reminded again of just how large the stakes are when you're a neurosurgeon. I'm reminded, too, of what the future holds for all of us. On the rare occasion that I have more than a few minutes to think about the patient who has just passed on, I also think about how that person reminds me of a family member or close friend.

In his final year of training, now abroad for a stint at New York-Presbyterian Hospital/Weill Cornell Medical Center, Parnia met a man whose death left an especially deep impression on him. Desmond Smith was a cheerful, gregarious West Indian immigrant, celebrating his sixty-second birthday at home just outside New York City. Despite a lifelong smoking habit, Smith was in good health and full of energy, until he began coughing up blood while preparing a big birthday breakfast. In the emergency room, he was still in good spirits, telling the twenty-two-year-old British medical student to cheer up, that everything would be fine. Smith did not seem gravely ill, so while they waited for a few test results, Parnia moved on to other patients.

Thirty minutes later, his pager was blaring the code for a cardiac arrest. Rushing back to the ER, he saw the tall figure of Desmond Smith sprawled on the floor, surrounded by a bustle of white coats. Smith never took another breath. Parnia was devastated and couldn't shake the questions that filled his head: How could a man so full of life be suddenly gone? What did *gone* really mean? Where was he now? Was this truly the end?

"I was left with the question of what did this person experience? Was he still with us in some way, or was he completely annihilated? I was fascinated, but I knew there was a science," said Parnia. "These questions in my mind made me want to investigate it myself."[5]

That hunger to understand never left, but Parnia's next three years were consumed with the grueling training of a medical residency. There was no time to pursue his curiosity about the possibility of life after death. So it was that three years went by until, the week after emerging as a newly minted, fully credentialed physician, Parnia sought out a doctor named Peter Fenwick, who was at the time perhaps the world's leading authority on near-death experience.

Fenwick is a neuropsychiatrist and neurophysiologist at King's College Hospital in London. In 1995, he had just published *The Truth in the Light,* an evaluation of more than three hundred near-death experiences. To some it might have seemed an odd obsession, but Parnia was fascinated. With Fenwick's encouragement, the young doctor started reading the scientific literature on near death. By 1997, he had landed a job at Southampton General Hospital in southern England, and he was ready to launch his own experiment.

At Southampton, Parnia won permission from the director to do a bit of interior decorating in the emergency rooms. When he described what he did, it struck me as one of the most fascinating experiments I've ever heard. He purchased 150 ceiling tiles, and at a local printer had one side of each tile coated with a unique image, like a photo or newspaper headline. With a bit of wire, he and some colleagues managed to hang all 150 tiles, image-side up, about two feet from the ceiling, in various spots around the emergency room and other areas that were used during emergency resuscitation. From the ground, the hanging panels just looked white, like regular ceiling tiles. But if anyone was really leaving their body to float around the room, they would be able to see the images.[6]

The study would include anyone who survived a cardiac arrest in the hospital. Sometime after being revived, they would be interviewed by Parnia or a fellow investigator and asked a simple question: "Do you remember anything from the period in which you were unconscious?" I think of it as trying to catch the white light in a bottle.

Over the next year, of sixty-three cardiac arrest survivors at Southampton Hospital, four answered yes to the question. The stories they told were interesting but didn't provide much insight into what might be the cause of NDEs. The first question Parnia wanted to answer was whether these people were really dying when they had their experience. Was there a difference physically in what happened to them as opposed to the other cardiac arrest patients? It turned out there was no significant difference in blood levels of oxygen, carbon dioxide, sodium, or potassium between the people who had NDEs and those who didn't. There was no particular difference in their religious beliefs, either, and nothing overtly religious about the experiences themselves. None of the four claimed to have left their body. And while it would have made for a much better story, none of them described seeing anything on the specially hung ceiling tiles.

The results were a bit of a letdown, but Parnia stood undaunted. He'd succeeded in bringing near-death research into the realm of science. Earlier investigators, like Moody and Kenneth Ring (who wrote *Lessons from the Light* and other NDE books), had been less rigorous, using loose definitions of death that lump Duane Dupre together with a cancer patient who has a vision while he lingers in the hospital, or a driver who sees her life flash before her eyes as she swerves to narrowly avoid an accident.[7]

By contrast, Parnia was studying people whose hearts had actually stopped, shutting off blood flow to the brain. A similar study, by Dr. Bruce Greyson, who founded the Division of Perceptual Studies at the University of Virginia, looked at people whose hearts were intentionally stopped for the purpose of implanting a defibrillator (to his dismay, none of them reported a near-death experience).[8] Now, you might say that having your heart stop is not quite the same thing as death. After all, anyone being interviewed afterward, for a study, has obviously managed to live through the experience. But Parnia was very comfortable playing with that line between life and death. In fact, he thought of death as a continuum and suspected that whether you were revived by CPR or died and stayed dead—well, those first few minutes were pretty much the same.

"Our roots began in the near-death experience, but what I talk about now is the 'actual death experience,'" Parnia told me. "We are actually objectively studying people during clinical death. As far as we can measure, there is no brain activity going on with these people. If that can be verified, it opens up a whole new field."

The pursuit of these questions is not always popular in the world of serious medicine. New York-Presbyterian Hospital/Weill Cornell Medical Center is the sister hospital of New York-Presbyterian Hospital/Columbia where Zeyad Barazanji was taken after his cardiac arrest. When my team first tried calling Parnia and said we wanted to ask about his near-death research, the public relations staff wouldn't put the call through.

He laughed when I finally reached him on the phone. "They've picked up on the negative connotations, and I've picked up on them, too. If you do a Google search, 99 percent of the available material is sort of out there. They don't want to be associated with that." Parnia knows the feeling—he was chagrined when his book on the subject, *What Happens When We Die,* ended up in the new age section of bookshops. "I thought to myself, 'Why is this sitting next to all these books about angels?'"

Indeed, most books and websites about near-death experience share an affinity for rainbow-hued skyscapes full of wispy clouds and sunbeams. Most people who have had a near-death experience, or who have thought about the topic at all, conclude that it's a sign of another spiritual world. Take, for instance, the experience of a woman I interviewed, a near-drowning victim. "I knew I was going to God. I knew I was going home. And I had no fear," said Jean Potter.[9]

Of course, the talk about meeting God unsettles people who think our lives are firmly grounded here in the physical universe. Nowhere in our lives is there as transparent an interface between spirituality and science as there is with near-death experience. But now a growing number of researchers, Parnia among them, are looking for a more standard medical explanation.

Some of these scientists suggest that a near-death experience is purely psychological, caused by intense fear or spiritual beliefs about death. Others say that it's essentially a hallucination caused by a critical lack of oxygen in the brain. For example, the tunnel that is such an integral part of many NDEs may simply be a narrowing of the visual field, just like the one someone experiences before they faint. In a fainting spell, it generally takes less than ten seconds for vision to disappear. This is caused by a lack of blood flow to delicate structures behind the eye that are needed for us to see.

What these theories have in common is the possibility that a mystical near-death experience has its basis in the nuts-and-bolts connections of the brain. I have been personally fascinated by the possibility that out-of-body experience may be grounded in brain circuitry. As I investigated this further, I realized the scientific precedent goes back at least to the 1930s. That's when the neuroscientist Wilder Penfield, who pioneered surgery to treat epilepsy, discovered that he could induce out-of-body experiences by stimulating certain parts of the brain with a metal probe.

A modern version of the experiment was written up

in 2007. Belgian neurologists reported in the *New England Journal of Medicine* that they had repeatedly induced out-of-body experiences by mechanically stimulating a part of the brain known as the superior temporal gyrus. The Belgians were trying to treat a debilitating case of tinnitus, or ringing in the ears. The treatment failed, but as they probed the brain to find the source of the problem, the doctors repeatedly caused their sixty-three-year-old patient to experience a sense of being outside his body. One episode lasted a full seventeen seconds.[10]

Confident they were on to something, the Belgians decided to take it a step further by performing specialized brain imaging tests. Remarkably, the scans taken during the procedure show two distinct areas of the brain suddenly lighting up: an area of the brain known as the temporoparietal junction, and more specifically the angular-supramarginal gyrus (associated with speech and self-perception, or sense of self); and the right precuneus and posterior thalamus (a brain region associated with the integration of the senses).

OUT-OF-BODY EXPERIENCES ARE actually pretty common. Even without direct brain stimulation, out-of-body experiences are reported by some epileptics, as well as by people under the influence of psychedelic drugs like PCP or ketamine—both of which are used legitimately as tranquilizers and illicitly as recreational drugs. A psychiatrist at the University of New Mexico, Rick Strassman, has actually theorized a direct role in NDE for another psychedelic drug, dimethyltryptamine (DMT). The brain naturally produces small amounts of DMT; Strassman suggests that in moments of intense bodily stress the pineal gland would release a larger amount of DMT, inducing the mystical near-death experience.[11]

Beyond drugs, some people are able to induce an out-of-body feeling through intense meditation or prayer. In case you are curious, the common link to all these things may be found in the brain's superior parietal lobe—found toward the rear on the top side of the head. I get asked all the time about which parts of the brain are responsible for different things. First off, it's easy to oversimplify, and keep in mind, the brain can change due to injury. And some people are just born with brains that don't obey the laws of anatomy texts.

But the superior parietal lobe does seem to be the home for out-of-body experiences. Two University of Pennsylvania neurologists have used brain scans to show how this might work. Dr. Andrew Newberg and Dr. Eugene D'Aquili say the superior parietal lobe is where we generate our sense of space and time; in subjects who were praying or meditating, the scans detected less blood flow to the area. In other words, that part of the brain was less active. Those test subjects felt less of a sharp distinction between themselves and the world around them. They were at one with their surroundings. It is easy to understand why these same two scientists started referring to the superior parietal lobe as the OAA, the orientation association area. It seems logical that a similar brain process in this area is responsible for out-of-body feelings experienced during an NDE.[12]

But then in 2006, Dr. Kevin Nelson, a neurologist at the University of Kentucky, proposed a different and novel explanation. Nelson is a tall and wiry man who still looks like a college student—except that the shock of bristling hair on his head is largely silver. He first became interested in near-death experience when he was doing his internship training in Albuquerque, New Mexico. One day, a man walked into the hospital and handed Nelson a small, beautiful painting. Nelson recognized a patient he had treated in the ICU, who had suffered a near-fatal cardiac arrest and only been released from the hospital a few days earlier. The man said the painting was a gift. He had made it himself and said it represented an experience he had had while lying in the ICU.[13]

"He came in with a really incredible story," says Nelson. "As he was lying there, the devil came to take his soul, but a guardian angel came to him, on his shoulder, and then along came Jesus Christ, his savior, who dispelled the devil—and at that point he knew he was no longer meant to leave this earth, and he almost immediately made a good recovery."

Nelson was glad to see the man doing well—he had grown to like him in the ICU—but he didn't put much stock in the story. "I was dismissive," says Nelson. "But I was struck by the intensity of his experience and how powerful it was. I kept the painting for years."

At the University of Kentucky in Lexington, Nelson is what's known as a neurophysiologist, specializing in treating muscle diseases like multiple sclerosis or myasthenia gravis. But even as he settled into his specialty, the same curiosity that nagged at Parnia started tugging on Nelson's sleeve. He found himself thinking more and more about the man who claimed that a guardian angel and Jesus had saved him from a heart attack. "In the back of my mind, I was thinking that not a single neurologist had ever paid attention to the phenomenon of near death," said Nelson. The brain must be central to the experience, he reasoned, just as it's central to any experience. And yet the only doctors who had taken the time to study NDEs were cardiologists or psychologists or even oncologists like Jeffrey Long, who runs the Near Death Experience Research Foundation (NDERF). Says Nelson, "These are not the neuroscientists who really know how the brain works."

Nelson closely read the first-person accounts in Moody's *Life After Life*, searching for clues the way a physician looks for clues in a patient's medical history. There was one account that particularly struck him. A woman was lying in a hospital's radiology suite, waiting for a scan of her liver, when she suffered a severe allergic reaction to a medication. She told Moody that she heard the radiologist walk over to a telephone on the wall, dial, and say, "Dr. James, I've killed your patient, Mrs. Martin." She struggled to let them know she was still alive but couldn't move a muscle. In this frozen manner, she watched and listened as an emergency team worked to revive her. She could see the needles going into her skin but couldn't feel them.[14]

Says Nelson, "She felt wide awake, and yet she was unable to move. I thought, what causes transient paralysis? Because that's what it sounds like, to a neurologist. I started thinking in terms of normal physical processes that cause paralysis, and what came to mind immediately was something we experience several times a night, and that's the REM stage of sleep. And then, many things started falling into place."

For Nelson, everything about an NDE—from the glowing light to the out-of-body experience to the mystical feeling—can be explained by a glitch in the body's sleep-wake machinery. More specifically, Nelson believes the near-death experience can be explained as a manifestation of a REM state—the same REM that we experience in deep sleep, when we dream.

Most people don't realize just how complex our sleep is, but anyone who's ever had trouble falling asleep, or struggled to drag themselves out of bed, can understand that sleep is more than a simple on-off switch. Healthy sleep involves multiple phases and multiple shifts in brain activity. Most of us have heard of REM sleep, named for the rapid eye movements—underneath the eyelids—that occur in this stage. In a healthy person, the REM stage makes up about 20 or 25 percent of total sleep time. The body and brain exhibit several distinctive changes. Aside from the eye movements, during REM sleep the body is paralyzed—a condition known as atonia. This is controlled by the brain, which during REM sleep stops releasing certain chemical transmitters, including serotonin and dopamine, which typically permit the muscles to be active.[15]

It's not uncommon for the gears of this machinery to get out of sync, so we're not completely awake or asleep at some given time. This can lead to some pretty weird behavior. Perhaps the most debilitating yet fascinating condition occurs when the REM stages break down and muscle paralysis doesn't occur. Sufferers may act out dreams or do bizarre things in their sleep, like trying to have sex or even lashing out with their fists. The condition is called REM behavior disorder. In severe cases, spouses have seriously injured each other or been forced to sleep in different beds for years. There was even an infamous case in Canada where a man named Kenneth Parks drove across town, broke into a house, and stabbed his wife's parents to death—all supposedly while asleep. Bizarre as it sounds, a jury acquitted Parks of murder, after hearing testimony that several members of his family suffered from extreme versions of REM behavior disorder.[16]

Aside from oddities like this, the REM stage is when we dream. Dreams, as we all know, can be unsettling, joyful, or terrifying—sometimes all in the same dream. But when thinking about that stunning bright light, it is important to know that the sights and sounds of our dreams are processed in parts of the brain that are different from the brain regions processing the sights and sounds we experience in our actual lives. For example, blind people are known to sometimes "see" things when they dream—especially if they've experienced sight at some point in their lives.[17]

What struck Nelson is that hearing about a near-death experience sounds a lot like someone telling you what they dreamed the night before. "If you listen to these near-death experiences, they're narratives—stories—and there's a plot. It's very action oriented. There's a lot of emotion, but very little language," says Nelson. That's the ineffability described by Moody. While some people can recount dreams in great detail, most of us have a lot of trouble describing just what happened in a dream. Time is slowed or distorted, and it's hard to remember the sequence of events. Once we awake, what's left is mostly a feeling—and maybe a few intense images. "If you're awake and kick in the dream machinery, the key brain parts are, number one, the limbic system, and two, the activation of the visual system. That's what really gets turned on when you're dreaming."

The limbic system is the network of brain structures that is involved in our emotions. It includes the hippocampus, which is vital to making new memories, and the amygdala, which not only plays a key role in memory, but is central to our stress response and its interplay with our emotions. According to Nelson, "Dreams are a play out of emotion more than anything else." It was sounding more and more as if sleep, dreams, and near-death experience were linked. According to the hypothesis, a near-death experience could be thought of as a sudden and powerful sleep episode interwoven with elaborate dreams.

If you want to try and find a scientific basis for an NDE, you also have to explain one of its cardinal features: the bright light—usually perceived in a sacred, awestruck manner. The "dead" person finds himself moving through a gloomy darkness, drawn inexorably to the brightness. Raymond Moody called this "the Being of Light" and wrote, "What is perhaps the most incredible common element in the accounts I have studied, and is certainly the element which has the most profound effect upon the individual, is the encounter with a very bright light" of "indescribable brilliance." According to Nelson, this can also be explained by a connection to REM sleep, because several studies have found increased activity in the brain's visual centers during the REM stage.

Nelson tested his hypothesis by interviewing fifty-five people who had reported a near-death experience. What he found is that people who have had an NDE are far more prone to REM intrusion than non-NDEers. Of the fifty-five "experiencers," thirty-three—60 percent—reported experiencing REM intrusion compared to just 24 percent of a control group. A participant was recorded as experiencing REM intrusion if they reported ever experiencing sleep paralysis, visual or auditory hallucinations around sleep, or cataplexy—sudden incidence of muscle weakness, which in extreme cases has been mistaken for death. One such sufferer—a woman named Allison Burchell—was famously taken to the morgue, while still alive, three times. NDEers are also eight times more likely to answer yes to the question "Just before falling asleep or awakening, have you had the sense that you are outside your body and watching yourself?"[18]

It's a small study and the results are not definitive, but

Nelson is confident he's cracked the code. The feeling of being dead would be caused by REM atonia—sleep paralysis. The tunnel and light would stem from loss of blood flow to the retina, combined with REM-stimulated visual imagery in the brain. The emotional aspects of the NDE would be fueled by the limbic system. An out-of-body feeling is common in the REM state and can also be triggered by stimulation of the same brain regions.

Nelson points out a few other things, as well. We know that a lack of oxygen can trigger an out-of-body reaction. Fighter pilots who experience blackouts or near blackouts from extreme g-forces—which block blood flow to the brain—often report intense dreams or dream imagery. There was also a 1994 study by a researcher who trained a bunch of college kids to hyperventilate and then suddenly stand up. Head rush, man! Not surprisingly, a fair number of the students reported brief blackouts; many also reported an out-of-body experience. I should also note that a life-threatening moment can be extremely stressful, and we know that stress can cause shortness of breath and perhaps a shortage of oxygen.

But here's something less obvious: stick your face into ice-cold water, and you will find yourself instantly gasping for breath. That's the diving reflex—sometimes referred to as the vagal reflex, named for the vagus nerve; it is so powerful that there are cases where people suffocated before they had a chance to drown after falling from a boat into icy waters.[19] The nerve can also be triggered by *emotional* stress. It sounds weird, but think about people who faint when they're extremely frightened—that's emotion triggering the vagal reflex.

Intriguingly, Nelson says you can trigger a REM-like state by stimulating that very same vagus nerve. This could help explain something that was nagging me before I heard his theory. People who go through a terrifying experience unharmed—such as someone who narrowly avoids a head-on highway collision—may also describe aspects of an NDE, like an out-of-body experience or a sense of time slowing down. Of course, all these NDEs and out-of-body experiences could just be the brain's protective reflex, a way to protect you from intense fear and stress. While the rest of your body is fighting for its life, your brain transports you to another place, full of bright tunnels and strong emotions.

Nelson's theory is fascinating, but it has raised a lot of hackles among other near-death researchers. After Nelson's study was published, Jeffrey Long and a therapist named Janice Miner Holden published a detailed thirty-five-page critique politely but firmly challenging every one of Nelson's conclusions.[20] Long (who had helped Nelson to recruit research subjects) is a radiation oncologist who runs one of the most prominent websites in the near-death community. Long says his Near Death Experience Research Foundation (NDERF) is a public service—he runs no advertising and takes no money for the work. According to Long, the NDERF website, nderf.org, receives more than fifty thousand unique visitors every month from more than twenty countries (Poles seem to take a special interest—there were 2,500 visitors from Poland alone the month we first spoke).

Over the years, more than 1,600 people have described their NDEs and taken the time to fill out an elaborate questionnaire.[21]

Long is a restless soul. Born and raised in Iowa, he says he's been licensed in ten different states over the past two decades. He moved to Albuquerque in early 2007 because he wanted to work with patients from the nearby Navajo territory. He traces his interest in NDEs to an article he stumbled across in 1986, by the Atlanta cardiologist and author Michael Sabom. "I was immediately fascinated. It should be impossible to be clinically dead and still have these lucid experiences," says Long. "I was astounded, and I remember vividly wondering, 'Why aren't more people studying this?'" He committed to doing the research himself after a drunken evening with a friend and his wife, where the wife told the story of an NDE she had had many years earlier—an experience where she coded on the operating table due to a severe allergic reaction; she says she floated away from her body, down the hall to a nursing station.

Long complains that Nelson's comparison group—the non-NDEers—is not typical; many are medical professionals and colleagues of Nelson. He also told me the research questionnaire was poorly designed and that Nelson fails to recognize dramatic differences between near-death experience and REM intrusion. For one thing, says Long, hallucinations stemming from REM intrusion—just before waking, or while falling asleep—are often "bizarre and unrealistic," such as seeing objects appear through cracks in a wall or movement in a painting on the wall. By contrast, says Long, memories from an NDE are lucid and rooted in the real world.

"NDEers almost uniformly don't say, 'Oh, that must have been a dream.' [On the website] we ask if they were conscious and alert, and about 75 percent say they were *more* alert, *more* conscious than normal," says Long. What's more, "there's a consistency of elements. This is not like a hallucination."

After hearing thousands upon thousands of NDEs, Long wonders, "Why do people 98 percent of the time encounter deceased relatives, as opposed to [their] dreams where it's common to encounter living people? We've even had people encounter deceased relatives who[m] they didn't know at the time were dead.... The totality of evidence shows there's something going on that's outside the medical evidence. NDEers almost always say, 'That wasn't a dream.' It was some different realm, some different aspect of their existence."

Long didn't really convince me that NDEs are evidence of another world. After all, my dreams can seem pretty realistic; often the only reason I know it was a dream is because when I wake up in bed the three-headed alligator or the tropical beach or the supermodel isn't there. But Long also raises another important point. REM intrusion—whether sleep paralysis or hallucinations—tends to be frightening or deeply unsettling. By contrast, most people who go through an NDE say the experience is almost supernaturally calm and peaceful, even joyful. Not only anecdotes, but real evidence does support this. In a 2001 study in the medical journal *The Lancet*, of sixty-two cardiac arrest patients who reported a near-death experience, more than half said the main emotions they experienced were "positive."[22] Long says these distinctive, positive emotions are powerful evidence that a near-death experience is not just REM intrusion in disguise.

An even fiercer critic of scientific NDE explanations is Dutch cardiologist Dr. Pim van Lommel—the author of that *Lancet* study. Now in his late sixties, van Lommel has the graying hair and kindly smile of a beloved family doctor. When he opens his mouth, though, he sounds like the commanding medical general who ran the cardiology ward of a major hospital in his native Holland. Even in English, his tone is clipped and certain. Like most physicians who study near-death experience, van Lommel traces his interest to an early patient—in his case, a man who was bitterly disappointed to be back among the living. Van Lommel says, "He told me about the tunnel, and the light, and music, and a beautiful landscape so beautiful that he was unhappy to be back in his body."[23]

Intrigued by the vivid story, van Lommel started asking his patients who survived a cardiac arrest if they remembered anything from the period of unconsciousness. Many did, and he began to analyze their accounts. His *Lancet* study looked at 344 cardiac arrest patients, only sixty-two of whom had what van Lommel categorized as a near-death experience. To van Lommel, this was proof that something was going on *outside* the body. "Our results show that medical factors cannot account for occurrence of NDE," he wrote. "Although all patients had been clinically dead, most did not have NDE. Furthermore, seriousness of the [physical] crisis was not related to occurrence or depth of the experience. If purely physiological factors caused NDE, most of our patients should have had this experience."

In the *Lancet*, van Lommel describes a signature case—a forty-four-year-old man, cyanotic and comatose, who had been discovered an hour earlier, lying unconscious in a meadow. He had no detectable heartbeat. To insert a breathing tube, van Lommel had to remove the man's dentures, which he placed on the crash cart in the medical bay. Only after defibrillation, "extensive" CPR, and ninety minutes of touch-and-go waiting was the patient stable enough to transfer to an intensive care unit.

A week later, the man was recuperating in the cardiac ward when van Lommel found him awake for the first time.

The moment he sees me he says: "Oh, that man knows where my dentures are." I am very surprised. Then he elucidates. "Yes, you were there when I was brought into hospital, and you took my dentures out of my mouth and put them onto that cart; it had all these bottles on it and there was this sliding drawer underneath and there you put my teeth." I was especially amazed because I remembered this happening while the man was in deep coma and in the process of CPR. When I asked further, it appeared the man had seen himself lying in bed, that he had perceived from above how nurses and doctors had been busy with CPR. He was also able to describe correctly and in detail the small room in which he had been resuscitated as well as the appearance of those present like myself. At the time that he observed the situation he had been very much afraid that we would stop CPR and that he would die.

Despite the man's poor initial prognosis, he was able to leave the hospital a month later. Wrote van Lommel, "He is deeply impressed by his experience and says he is no longer afraid of death."

Van Lommel argues forcefully for the view that NDEs prove the existence of an unseen world, a level of consciousness beyond the confines of the brain. In a 2007 article, he writes, "Because of the occasional and verifiable out-of-body experiences, like the one involving the dentures in our study, we know that the NDE must happen *during* the period of unconsciousness, and *not* in the first or last seconds of cardiac arrest. So we have to come to the *surprising conclusion* that during cardiac arrest NDE is experienced during a loss of all functions of the cortex and of the brainstem."[24] (van Lommel's italics)

A lot of people find this convincing. It certainly tackles a question that arises from the most dramatic stories, where a patient seems to have accurate memories from a time when he or she was measurably, clinically dead. There are thousands of stories like this, but it's extremely rare to find one that comes with medical documentation. Probably the best-known case involves a woman named Pam

Reynolds, a Juilliard-trained singer and songwriter who lives just outside Atlanta. In 1991, Reynolds was working with her family's record business, writing her own songs and also raising five children when she received alarming news—she'd been diagnosed with an aneurysm of the basilar artery, a major blood vessel in the brain. Doctors told Reynolds it could rupture at any time and advised surgery to fix the damaged artery.[25]

Because of the aneurysm's size and location, the operation would be unusually complicated. The aneurysm was large and fragile, on a major artery, pulsing with blood every second. Any repair work would run an extremely high risk of popping the artery open by mistake; the blood loss would likely be immediate, massive, and fatal. Given the danger, Reynolds' doctors planned a relatively new type of operation, cooling her body from its normal temperature of 98.6 degrees Fahrenheit to just 60 degrees. Her breathing would stop. Blood flow would slow to a trickle. Brain activity—on a standard EEG monitor—would be unnoticeable. To the casual eye, she would be dead.

The operation in August 1991 went as planned—a perfect success. But when Reynolds awoke, she had an amazing story to tell. While not in pain, she had been conscious during every step of the procedure. She had felt surgeons drill through her skull with an electric saw ("The noise was awful, like the drill in a dentist's office"), then floated out of her head and watched the operation from above.[26]

She found herself in the presence of her late grandmother. There was no sound, but Reynolds knew somehow that her grandmother was calling her—down a tunnel that wasn't quite a tunnel, toward a pinprick of light that kept getting bigger and bigger. In that place of light, she found herself surrounded by deceased relatives, who fed and nurtured her. She was warned not to go farther, because she wouldn't have a way to get back. Though drawn by the light, Reynolds thought of her family at home and agreed to return. Her late uncle led her back to the tunnel, and she found herself looking down once more at:

> ...the thing—my body. It looked terrible, like a train wreck. It looked like what it was: dead....It scared me and I didn't want to look at it.
>
> It was communicated to me that it was like jumping into a swimming pool. No problem, just jump right into the swimming pool. I didn't want to, but I guess I was late or something because he [the uncle] pushed me. I felt a definite repelling and at the same time a pulling from the body. The body was pulling and the tunnel was pushing....It was like diving into a pool of ice water....It hurt!
>
> When I came back, they were playing "Hotel California" and the line was "You can check out anytime you like, but you can never leave."

Michael Sabom, the researcher who first inspired Jeffrey Long, wrote an account of Reynolds' case, which became a sensation. She's easily the most-cited example of a person having memories at a time when they were "clinically dead." The thing is, even the term clinically dead is open to interpretation. In the United States, we use EEG or brain monitoring to declare there is no brain activity—that someone is dead. Transplant surgeons wait for this proof before removing organs, but to an extent, that's arbitrary. In Japan, it's only after heart activity is stopped on an EKG that someone is considered dead. Brain death versus cardiac death. Nelson, who has not reviewed Reynolds' medical records, seriously doubts that she truly had no electrical brain activity throughout the operation.

Nelson speculates that Reynolds might have been partially awake for at least part of the operation, despite the anesthesia. So-called "anesthesia awareness" isn't as rare as you might think. According to the American College of Anesthesiologists, 1 or 2 percent of all surgical patients experience at least partial awareness during their operation. This number is for surgeries where the patient is actually supposed to be knocked out; it doesn't include operations done under local anesthesia or other cases where the patient is intentionally left conscious. Here's an interesting aside: the brain is totally free of pain receptors. In fact, in certain brain operations the patient is left awake so he or she can communicate with surgeons during the operation to ensure that no tissue is removed that would affect the patient's ability to talk or other skills. Of course, it may be that none of this is relevant to the case of Pam Reynolds or any NDEer, but it's not far-fetched to think that a patient might be partially conscious even during an invasive brain operation.

Some cases of anesthesia awareness are horror stories where the patient suffers intense pain from the surgeon's knife but is paralyzed and can't cry out. This version was dramatized in the 2007 Hollywood thriller *Awake*; its publicists said it would do for anesthesia what *Jaws* did for sharks. In other cases, the pain medication portion of the cocktail does work, leaving the patient calm and numb—but still aware, at least partially aware, of their surroundings. Nelson started thinking about a connection between anesthesia awareness and NDEs because of a quirk in his survey results: four of the fifty-five subjects who reported near-death experiences also said they were awake during surgery.[27]

As I continued my discussions with experts around the world, I realized a possibility: that it all comes down to memory. Biologically there's no physical difference between "real" memories and memories of something that never actually happened. Listening to Nelson, I was reminded of research done by Harvard psychologist Richard McNally and his students. McNally's specialty is memory, especially the way it can be distorted. He's done extensive work on false memories, and his work on how easy it is to produce false memories—through suggestion—has strongly influenced the way that courts handle testimony about old, supposedly repressed memories.

One big question is whether the brain forms and stores false memories any differently from the way it handles real memories. To try and answer this, McNally's then-student Susan Clancy wanted to examine memories that almost certainly were not based in reality. She decided to interview people who claimed to have been abducted by space aliens. Their stories were eerily alike, full of gray-headed aliens with big eyes, taking people aboard spacecraft for medical or sexually themed experiments. Clancy came to an interesting conclusion: she decided that the memories were real, even if the abductions were not. The mechanism for producing these memories, in Clancy's view, was sleep paralysis. The people had only dreamed about being abducted, but the dreams were so vivid—complete with an intense physical feeling of being unable to move while being examined by aliens—that they were convinced it really happened.[28]

Kevin Nelson says the same about near-death experience. "I don't think it's inaccurate recall, although I do think that recall and memory at a time when your brain is potentially impaired by low oxygen or low blood sugar might be called into question," he says. "When we're dreaming, the fascinating thing is we don't know we're dreaming. There are rare exceptions called lucid dreams, but for the vast majority of people, we don't have that insight. The brain turns it off normally."

There's reason to think that memory of NDEs is even less reliable than memories of a dream. For one thing, memory is often the first thing to go when the brain is running out of oxygen. The seat of memory is the CA1 region of a brain structure called the hippocampus. According to Larry Squire of the University of California at San Diego, a neuroscientist and expert on memory, when cells of the CA1 region are deprived of oxygen, they go into an overwrought metabolic state, burning energy at a frantic pace.[29] "They basically fire themselves to death over a period of a few days," explains Squire. "These patients end up with memory loss." To be blunt, you can't trust the memory of someone whose brain was oxygen deprived, even for a short time.

Less obvious but equally true is the fact that memory is distorted by stress. Under stress, the body releases certain hormones, like cortisol, which trigger activity in the amygdala. The amygdala is about the size and shape of an almond. It plays a vital role in transforming short-term memories into long-term ones. When there's too much activity, the process is impaired. This means that under stressful conditions, people are far less likely to recall the details occurring around them. This has major real-world implications. For example, memory experts say that eyewitness testimony is extremely unreliable, even if courts and juries have been slow to recognize this.

Many people mistakenly think their memory of a stressful event is excellent. That's because the emotional aspect of the memory is so strong. This also goes back to the amygdala. Along with helping the memory process, the amygdala plays a key role in the limbic system—the system we talked about earlier that regulates our emotions. Stress might keep us from remembering the details, but we never forget how we *felt* at certain times, whether it's a first kiss or a firefight in Baghdad. Post-traumatic stress disorder is essentially a memory problem; the terrifying aspects of an experience are seared in the victim's mind, a painful memory that gets stronger each time it's recalled.[30]

So what does all this have to do with NDEs? Well, a life-threatening emergency can be pretty frightening. Even if you don't panic, it's hard to imagine a more emotionally charged situation. If we think about memory under stress, it's easy to see how people might vividly recall the experience, even if they don't accurately remember all the details. The details of NDE accounts seem especially shaky in a case where the patient was not only stressed out, but oxygen deprived and maybe even pumped full of powerful medication.

If this casts doubt on the reality of NDEs, it also seems to pose a challenge to the scientific explanations. Let's say you did have a dreamlike experience. How would you remember it when you were in cardiac arrest and your brain had no oxygen?

Here's the thing: A memory, even of a real event, isn't a perfect snapshot that we've filed away. It's a puzzle of different parts—sights, sounds, emotional content, and other details. Each time the memory is recalled, the different parts of the puzzle are called up and patched together, and each time the memory is remade, the connections in the brain are reinforced and the memory gets stronger. The problem is, it isn't always accurate. Each memory is, in a sense, being rebuilt from scratch every time, and new puzzle pieces can get thrown in by mistake—or even on purpose. Countless experiments show that it's incredibly easy to induce false memories by making a few simple suggestions. In the same way, a real memory can be distorted by suggestion after the fact—for example, a vague memory of darkness and light might over time become a vivid memory of a tunnel, as the story is told again and again. [31]

Another distortion that might be relevant to NDEs involves time. Unless there are specific cues to prompt us, we often remember events as happening in a different order than they really did. It's possible that Pam Reynolds accurately remembered part of a conversation among her doctors, but inaccurately recalled that it took place while she was "dead," when in fact they were talking a few minutes before she became unconscious.

One thing that's clear: whether or not near-death experiences are real, they usually have a profound effect on the people who have them. This holds true whether someone nearly dies under carefully recorded conditions in a hospital or in a setting where the person merely came close to physical harm.

Pam Wedding, now sixty-two, was a nineteen-year-old student at the University of Georgia when she agreed to go white-water rafting with a friend named Jim.[32] Wedding loved to spend time hiking and camping, but she wasn't an experienced rafter. Nevertheless, she and Jim launched their boat on a section of the Ocoee River that was favored by expert kayakers. Making matters worse, there had been heavy rains the night before. Almost immediately after pushing off into the water, they lost their paddles and found themselves in serious trouble. Holding on for dear life, Wedding and Jim rode the river around a bend, past a large, rocky outcrop. Says Wedding, "I saw these people waving. That's what I thought at first. But they were really saying, 'Go back!' "

She soon could see why. Over the roar of the river she made out an even louder sound. It was water spilling over a low-head dam, dangerous in any circumstance, since the water falling over the edge forms what rafters call a hydraulic, a circular current of water going back toward the dam face. Worse for Wedding and her friend, the swollen river had actually broken off a portion of the dam, causing a powerful current that had them hurtling straight for the gap.

"I went into some kind of shock. I remember [Jim] saying 'Hold on!' The funny thing is—I wasn't scared. I was just, you know, holding on," she said. The roar of the river faded in her ears as the boat shot over the edge of the dam. Caught in the hydraulic, Wedding could barely move a muscle against the powerful current that held her, churning, underwater.

"I just stayed under, and when I went down, it was just dark. Just dark," she recalls. I would imagine an unbelievably terrifying experience, but Wedding says she felt no sense of panic. Time seemed to slow, and each thought came to her as clear as crystal. "I was thinking, very clearly, 'It's dark and I'm underwater.' And I said, 'Okay, I'm gonna breathe in.' And I could breathe in, and I could breathe out, and I thought, 'Well, this can't be happening, because I can't breathe in the water. And so I thought I was dead.'

"And then I started to get these little vignettes coming in. I saw myself there as a young child, with my father who died when I was seven and a half, and with my brother, who's still alive." The images drifted by, and a sense of peace filled her body. "It was just holy, absolute peace," she said.

To be clear, Wedding may have been in grave danger but she certainly wasn't near death from a physical standpoint. She wasn't even unconscious. She did experience a feeling of intense clarity and a sense that time had slowed. Kevin Nelson suggests that this bodily reaction to danger may be an evolutionary adaptation, akin to the fight-or-flight response that may immediately precede it. Says Nelson, "You have to calm down in order to take appropriate action. If you hear a lion's roar or you spot a lion, you have to find a tree to climb." You can't do that if you're in a state of panic. "You can't be looking all over. You have to focus on your escape route."

When we find ourselves in danger, a brain center called the locus coeruleus releases adrenaline, which makes us more alert and gives us a jolt of energy. When the neurons of the locus coeruleus are firing fast, we're highly aroused. When they slow down, we're calmer and more focused on the task.[33] That's old news to neurologists, but Nelson sees a new twist. You see, in animal experiments, the only time the neurons of the locus coeruleus stop firing completely is during REM sleep. If Nelson's theory is right, the high stress of a near-death situation triggers REM stage, which leads to the overwhelming sense of peace and clarity found in NDEs. It's a tantalizing connection. Nelson admits he's going out on a limb, but if he's right, it might explain the common threads between true NDEs and other similar experiences.

Pam Wedding saw the light—a classic near-death experience. "There was the light they always talk about," she continued her story. "A light just started seeming like it was coming from in front of me, filling up the space. It was just so beautiful, so inviting. I just knew that whatever it was, it was all good.

"I thought, 'It's okay. I'm dead, and it's going to be fine.' And then, somebody just grabbed me around the waist. A hand came around my waist and pulled upward, and I just shot up. And when I reached the surface, there was Jim, my friend, pulling me over to the side."

The experience was too overwhelming to describe at the time, so Wedding didn't say anything about it when she crawled out of the water. She and Jim just asked each other if they were okay, nodded, pulled out the boat, and went home. Though they stayed in touch after college, they didn't discuss the incident for more than thirty years, until Jim was visiting Atlanta for the 1996 Summer Olympics. Over dinner, Wedding mentioned to Jim's teenage son that his dad was a hero for pulling her out of the water. Jim just stared at her across the table. At first, she thought he didn't know what she was talking about, and then he spoke. Quietly he said he didn't pull her up but just helped her to the side of the river once she was free of the churning hydraulic. He said, "We thought you were dead. And then you literally came flying out of the water!"

I asked if maybe it wasn't just the action of the spinning water, throwing her to safety. No, she was certain. "I know it sounds crazy, but a hand grabbed my wrist and pulled me out of the water," says Wedding. "On some level I thought maybe it was my father [who had died twelve years before].

I swear, as much as I'm sitting here, I felt that happen, like 'You're not ready to go anywhere!' "

The trigger of an NDE doesn't seem to matter when it comes to the long-term impact. It doesn't seem to matter whether physical death actually occurrs for a few seconds or minutes or if the person simply undergoes a terrifying experience, like going over a waterfall and being held underwater for a few minutes. The near-death experience has a profound effect. Several long-term studies document that most people who report an NDE emerge with a sense of knowledge or enlightenment. One NDEer who suffered a near-fatal heart attack told me that even though he's not religious, he returned to life with a sense that he had just received a message—"I just don't know what it is."[34]

According to Jeffrey Long, this sense of meaning doesn't happen overnight. In fact, he says the changes in personality and outlook take seven years on average to reach their peak. And sometimes longer. Pam Wedding spent most of her adult life in the corporate world, but shortly after discussing the near-drowning incident for the first time—thirty-one years after it happened—she traveled to Tibet, became a Buddhist, and started volunteering at a hospice, where she continues to this day.

Pam Reynolds certainly felt a transformation. On her website, Reynolds writes that she no longer has a fear of death and that she's become so "sensitive" that going out in large crowds makes her feel uncomfortable. She feels more compassion and understanding for others: "I'm slow to anger and I have the patience of Job."

Pim van Lommel reinterviewed his study participants two years after their cardiac arrests, and again six years after that. At both junctures, people who went through an NDE were less afraid of death, more likely to believe in the afterlife, more likely to say they understood the purpose of life, and more likely to appreciate "ordinary things." What's more, their questionnaires showed them to be more "loving" and "empathetic"; more involved with their families; and ranking higher on measures of understanding others, sensing inner meaning, and showing their own feelings.[35] A skeptic might say that people who are most likely to report an NDE are the same people who might already be interested in the afterlife and to feel empathy toward others. Fair enough, but in study after study, similarly dramatic results have been found.

Long says these transformations generally happen only when a person believes that what they experienced while "dead" was real. He says, "They know there's some different realm, some different aspect of their existence. That's why they have the changes. They don't fear death. They know there's an afterlife, and they think it's wonderful. You just have to listen to them." Long's biggest beef with mainstream researchers, he says, is that scientists like Nelson miss the main point: that to truly understand what's going on, you need to listen to the experiences.

Still, Long doesn't dismiss the REM hypothesis, and he's eager to see it tested by a definitive study. That would certainly be a monumental task. At a major hospital or hospitals, anyone entering over the course of a year would be asked a set of detailed questions to determine if they would qualify for a diagnosis of REM intrusion disorder. Meanwhile, anyone who suffered a cardiac arrest while in the hospital would be quizzed about whether they'd had a near-death experience—and asked to describe it in detail. If it turns out that people who report REM intrusion beforehand are more prone to a near-death experience, that would support Nelson's theory. Fascinating, but it seems unlikely that any such study will be done in the foreseeable future.

Pim van Lommel insists that the true explanation for NDEs lies outside the brain. Our brains, in his view, don't produce consciousness but tune in to an outside, preexisting consciousness found in electromagnetic fields all around us. He believes that people who experience an NDE are somehow able to bring in the signal, even as their own brain ceases to function.[36] "I think that death is another kind of consciousness, a change of the level of consciousness, like Buddha said," says van Lommel. "Death is death of the physical body, but not the end of the essence you are. You have your consciousness, and that remains."

In mainstream medical circles, this theory is controversial to say the least, but van Lommel is supremely confident. In a 2007 paper, he wrote that it is "inevitable" to conclude that consciousness and the brain are separate and that this understanding "might well induce a huge change in the scientific paradigm in western medicine."[37]

In 2008, Sam Parnia finally launched what he hopes will be a more definitive experiment, involving more than two dozen major medical centers in the United States and Europe.[38] Much like his earlier work in Southampton, Parnia's researchers are asking patients who survive a cardiac arrest what they remember of the experience. Parnia wants to determine once and for all whether it's possible for the mind to continue to function, even when the brain no longer does. He thinks the new study will go a long way toward pinning down what's really going on with these lights, tunnels, and out-of-body experiences.

"I'm still very skeptical about the whole thing, but until we can verify these things objectively, we can't say they don't happen," says Parnia. "Is it a false memory? My personal view [is] that probably that's what we'll find. But if we find that mind and human consciousness could be separate, that people somehow see things from the ceiling, then we have an amazing discovery."

Nearly dying was a spark for Duane Dupre. He left the stressful work of managing supermarkets to focus on spending more time with his four grandchildren and doing good works. Along with ten of his pals, Dupre started a foundation called Ten Friends Cooking, which caters big events and gives all the proceeds to charity. He knows what he saw while he was dead and says he knows it was a miracle, even if he isn't quite sure what happened to him: "People say you must have been dreaming. You must have just imagined it. And maybe they're right. We'll see."

CHAPTER FIVE

What Lies Beneath

*No event is so terribly well adapted to inspire the
supremeness of bodily and of mental distress, as is
burial before death.... What I have now to tell is of
my own actual knowledge—of my own positive and
personal experience.*

—Edgar Allan Poe, "The Premature Burial"

D R. MARK RAGUCCI was so far gone, his doctors thought
he'd never come back. For nearly two months after
a surgery that went badly awry, Ragucci was completely
unresponsive, dead to the world in his hospital bed. "They
said I had irreparable brain damage from having no oxygen
to my brain," he recalls. "They said I showed no response
to stimuli. That means they could shine a light in my eyes,
poke me with a needle, whatever, it wouldn't register. I was
a vegetable."[1]

For two months he lay in a darkened room while his
mother, father, and wife kept vigil, all waiting for a miracle.
The head of the unit, a physician with an elite medical education and more than a decade of experience in one of the

country's top hospitals, told them to forget it. So did two other doctors with the combined weight of half a century of medical experience. The doctors in the crisp white coats, the medical literature on which they relied, all gave his family the same simple message: pull the plug.[2]

Up to this point, we've been talking about death as stoppage of the heart. That's been the meaning of death almost as long as humans have been around. But in an American hospital today, that's not what doctors mean by death: They're talking about whether the brain can function in a meaningful way, about whether consciousness is irretrievably lost. They're talking about brain death. And here, the line between life and death is shifting just as much, if not more, as it is for the doctors who try and keep our hearts beating and the blood pumping through our veins.

You won't find a better example than Ragucci. His doctors might have given up, but he can tell the story today because one doctor didn't—and because something inside Ragucci was able to bounce back, something that gave him the strength to cheat death: brain death.

The concept of brain death first gained popularity among a small group of surgeons in the 1950s. They were transplant surgeons, intent on taking body parts from a patient with no hope of survival and giving them to one who might be saved. Through the 1950s and most of the 1960s, these surgeons made tremendous technical advances toward the removal and implantation of kidneys, hearts, and livers in animals. But except for the use of a single kidney—which could be removed without killing the donor—they were forbidden from trying human transplants. No hospital would allow a body part to be removed from an organ donor until the patient's heart stopped beating on its own. Any doctor who defied these guidelines might be prosecuted for murder. Of course, once the heart stops, tissues throughout the body begin to die, so the restriction against taking organs from a living body meant that surgeons were limited to using organs damaged by the lack of oxygen. In leading hospitals, surgeons would hover around a dying man or woman, anxiously watching the monitor that would tell them when his or her heart stopped, so the transplant operation could begin. Not surprisingly, survival rates in early transplant cases were poor.

The tide began to turn in 1967 when Dr. Christiaan Barnard, a South African surgeon, convinced South Africa to pass legislation allowing two neurosurgeons to declare a patient brain-dead if the brain showed no detectable activity. That legal victory helped Barnard find the donor he needed to perform the first human heart transplant in December of that year.[3] In 1970, Kansas became the first U.S. state to recognize the concept of brain death, and others quickly followed. The legal change was hastened along by the sensational trial of pioneering heart surgeon Dr. Richard Lower, who was hit with murder charges in Virginia after transplanting the heart of a brain-dead donor. He was acquitted in 1972, and the case was followed by a loosening of legal restrictions around the country. Even now, some countries—including Japan—cling to a definition of death based primarily on stoppage of the heart.[4] But not the United States. If you're an American watching over a critically ill relative, it's more likely you will hear that they are brain-dead than that their heart has quit beating.

The thing is, brain death isn't always easy to figure out. There's a range of similar diagnoses, from a vegetative state to simply saying that a patient is in a deep coma. Most coma patients are measured with the Glasgow Coma Scale, which gauges alertness, responsiveness to stimuli, and the ability to communicate. The scale runs from 3 to 15, with 15 being normal consciousness and 3 being total unresponsiveness. At his low point, Ragucci was a 3.

Many patients with such severe damage don't make it out of the hospital. Those who survive almost always emerge with catastrophic disabilities, like permanent man-in-a-barrel syndrome or the total loss of speech. Many patients never truly wake up, although they may progress to a stage where they sleep and wake on a regular cycle, even as they display no awareness of themselves or of their surroundings. A good example, according to her doctors, was Terri Schiavo, the woman who in 2005 reignited the debate about the definition of death. Patients like Schiavo may move muscles or even open and move their eyes, but the movements are simple reflexes. This is known as a vegetative state.[5] You might have heard of a persistent vegetative state or a permanent vegetative state; this is exactly what it sounds like: doctors see no hope of getting better.

A notch higher on the scale is something called a minimally conscious state. This diagnosis was only formalized in 2002, as researchers grasped for more fine-tuned distinctions. A person in a minimally conscious state may appear vegetative most of the time but show occasional glimmers of awareness. They might demonstrate "intent," the ability to plan movements; they might remember new information; they might track objects with their eyes or even make efforts to communicate.

Non-doctors often use the phrase brain dead interchangeably with these other conditions, but true brain death is something else. It means that not only higher brain areas are wiped out, but also the brain stem, which is the seat of functions like breathing and heartbeat. A patient who is brain-dead cannot survive without complete mechanical support of their breathing and circulation. Another thing about brain death: We've been taught that it's final. Patients don't get better. Someone who is brain-dead isn't really a person anymore; they're a vessel preserving the individual organs.

Each diagnosis—brain death, vegetative state, minimally conscious state—is a crucial and yet often blurry marker on the landscape of consciousness. Making matters even more complicated, a patient may improve or decline from one state to another. It's exceedingly hard to tell whether a particular patient might or might not get better, even though the very language of the diagnosis—"permanent," "perpetual"—suggests a degree of certainty.

The average person peering into the hospital room would have a hard time telling the difference between a brain-dead patient and someone in a persistent vegetative state, or even a minimally conscious state. More alarming, many doctors, even trained neurologists, can't tell the difference either. One study of patients in nursing homes found that of those who were diagnosed as being in a persistent or permanent vegetative state, about one in three actually became fully conscious within a year. Joseph Fins, a physician who oversees ethical consults and end-of-life care at New York-Presbyterian Hospital/Weill Cornell Medical Center, says the field is crying out for better diagnostic methods: "It's a situation we would find intolerable anywhere else, to have a third of all the patients misdiagnosed."[6]

Although his specialty is internal medicine, not neurology, Fins has taken—almost by accident—a leading role in the medical debate over how to measure consciousness and the odds of recovery. For nearly two decades, Fins has sat on the ethics committee of Weill Cornell Medical Center. The committee meets to discuss all sorts of complicated cases—for example, a little more than a decade ago, Fins was confronted with the case of a patient who had advanced metastatic cancer. Pressure from the tumor had forced the patient into a coma, and her doctors were unsure how much they should do to ensure that the woman did not suffer. Pain-relieving drugs like morphine are dangerous in high doses because they depress the respiratory system, so it's considered safer to withhold them. On the other hand, doctors would never do that to a conscious patient, because the pain might be unbearable.

"The question was, 'Should we treat this patient's pain?'" Fins recalls. "Could they perceive their pain?" Fins realized he had no idea what the answer was. While considering the case, he recognized a neurologist named Nicholas

Schiff in line at the hospital cafeteria. Fins didn't know him well, but Schiff had a reputation as someone who thought about these things. "So I asked Nico to write a commentary [for *The Journal of Pain Management*]," said Fins. "And that was the beginning of a beautiful relationship."

Schiff had been interested in consciousness for a long time. His mentor was Dr. Fred Plum, the neurologist who first coined the phrase "vegetative state" back in 1972.[7] Today, Schiff is one of the hottest names in medicine; in late 2007, he was named one of *Time* magazine's one hundred most influential people. He's seen his share of shocking recoveries.

Most famously, in 2006, Schiff examined the brain of an Arkansas man who had woken up after nearly two decades in a coma. Terry Wallis was nineteen years old, with a five-month-old daughter, when his pickup truck veered off the side of a steep hill. Along with causing severe brain damage, the accident left him completely paralyzed. Nineteen years later, a nursing-home aide, making conversation, asked who was coming to visit that day. The aide's jaw dropped as Wallis answered, "Mom." Within months, he was speaking frequently and had even regained the ability to make new memories.[8] His family allowed Schiff to peer inside Wallis' brain, using PET scans and diffusion tensor imaging. He found that Wallis had grown new brain connections, working around the severe damage he suffered in the crash.[9] That's pretty surprising to many people; until recently most doctors were taught in medical school that brain cells, once dead, do not regenerate.

As it stands now, neither brain imaging nor standard clinical exams are very reliable as far as determining a coma patient's true level of consciousness, much less how likely it is they'll get better.[10] Looking at behavior or looking at what brain parts are damaged—that only scratches the surface. It doesn't tell you what the neurons are doing. In the meantime, hospitals and insurance companies don't have the time to wait for answers. It's pretty alarming when you think about it. "You see people all the time," says Schiff. "They're three weeks out from the injury; they've got one week left on your standard thirty-day stay that you get with modern insurance. And the diagnosis between minimally conscious state and vegetative state might make the difference between staying in the hospital for treatment and going to a nursing home."

Fins weighs in: "In the old days, it was almost easier. The doctor would come out and say, 'There's no hope.' But today, it's more complicated. These pronouncements need to be evidence based."

We do know a few things. It turns out that two factors are especially important when it comes to determining the odds: one is how long a person has been in a coma; perhaps even more important is how they got there in the first place. A patient who lost blood flow to the brain because of a stroke or cardiac arrest generally fares worse than someone with a traumatic brain injury, like what you would get from a car accident or a blow to the head. The reason isn't complicated: an injury might damage only parts of the brain, whereas a loss of oxygen will damage every single cell. Terry Wallis was injured in a car accident. However, after suffering a cardiac arrest and going without oxygen to his brain for at least five minutes, Zeyad Barazanji was at an even higher risk.

ON THE EIGHTH floor of New York-Presbyterian Hospital/ Columbia University Medical Center, Barazanji lay senseless, surrounded by tubes, oblivious to the glorious view of the Hudson River from just across the hall. The sliding glass doors could not keep the space from feeling cramped; almost every last inch was taken up by the bed and the stacks of machinery beside it. The one exception was the chair on which Barazanji's wife, Raoua, sat silently holding her husband's hand.

It had been nearly a week since he arrived in the unit, taken by ambulance in the dead of night from another hospital bed less than two miles away. He hadn't stirred when paramedics drove under the high arching stone above the ambulance arrival zone or when his stretcher was jolted out of the ambulance's back and wheeled through the quiet hospital lobby. Settled in his room on the eighth floor, he wasn't stirring at all.[11]

Although his eyes were closed and there was no obvious indication that a spirit flickered behind them, the rest of his body had been the site of a raging battle for several hours. Barazanji's skull had a hairline crack where his head had struck the side of the treadmill from which he fell. Between that blow and the lack of oxygen from his cardiac arrest, the cells and tissues of his body were bruised and swelling in agitated response—most alarmingly, in his brain.

For Raoua Barazanji,[12] it was terrifying. Her husband lay as if asleep, pale machines and tubing bristling, it seemed, from every inch of skin. She could read the concern on the faces of the doctors who stopped by his bedside. Dr. Stephan Mayer had started Barazanji on the non-FDA approved hypothermia. Cooling pads were wrapped around Barazanji's arms and legs, and he was strapped into what looked like a padded vest—each compartment filled with cold liquid, cooling the fire that raged in every tissue of his body. Old cells would need to heal; new ones would need to grow. It would take energy and time. The cooling would help buy that time.

Mayer had promised Raoua and the patient's niece that he would try everything, but even Mayer was not optimistic. Like many patients whose brain goes without oxygen for an extended period of time, Barazanji's brain was being rattled by seizures. It was frightening to watch the normally calm professor's body being wracked by uncontrollable shakes. Soon these seizures were coming every few minutes. It was quickly becoming a life-threatening condition called status epilepticus.

Status epilepticus is the uncontrolled firing of neurons in the brain. Our nervous system is made of neurons, forming the grid that carries all the information that our brains send out and receive, whether it's working out a math equation, telling a finger muscle to start wiggling, or feeling pain when that finger is pricked. The signals are transmitted across synapses, minute gaps between the neurons. An electrical charge causes the release of chemicals that bridge the gap. To function, neurons require a brief period of rest to recharge the supply of chemicals. In a brain gripped by seizures, that rest never comes. Unchecked, the condition is a death spiral. A brain that's continually seizing is constantly burning fuel, burning energy. As a rule of thumb, if status epilepticus continues for more than an hour, neurons start to die and the patient with them.

To stop the electrical frenzy, to keep the brain circuits from burning themselves out, the Columbia physicians gave Barazanji a massive dose of the sedative propofol. Over the course of an hour, the brain waves on the EEG monitor turned from a spiking, storm-driven sea to shorter, gently rolling swells. Barazanji was in a deep, medically induced coma. As Dr. Mayer, the chief neurologist, explained it to Raoua, sedation along with the cold was just like wrapping the brain in cotton to let it heal. The neurons would have a chance to rest, a chance to recharge and recover. Or so they hoped.

IT WAS ON this same floor, five years earlier, that Mayer met the patient who forced him to rethink his whole approach to neurointensive care. Mayer first heard about Mark Ragucci when he got a call from Ragucci's wife, Laura. A doctor like her husband, she crisply laid out the situation. Mark had already been in a coma for more than two weeks at another New York hospital. The physicians there, she said, were "laying the crepe," as doctors sometimes say about cases deemed hopeless. The family wasn't happy. They wanted to give Mark every possible chance of survival. Moved by the strength of the request, Mayer agreed to take a look.

"We did something in our unit that we never ordinarily do," said Mayer. "Usually, we only transfer patients from other hospitals if we think there's something we could do to help them that they can't get at their present hospital." Mayer paused. "In this case, we really didn't think we had anything to offer."

Although he agreed to take the case, Mayer privately agreed with the assessment of the other neurologists. He too thought that if Ragucci somehow made it out of the hospital, he would live out his days in a futile, eyes-open coma. Beyond the grim clinical picture, Ragucci's MRI images were the clincher. A healthy brain scanned by MRI looks like a symmetrical sculpture of grays and black. On Ragucci's scan, there were half a dozen large white blotches scattered around the picture. Two of them lay just two inches behind his eyes, the largest about the size of a quarter. Ragucci had holes all over his brain. Each white blotch was dead tissue, the cells burst open, destroyed by a lack of oxygen. For a neurologist, the writing was on the wall. The patient would not survive without never-ending artificial respiration and a feeding tube. Not a life that anyone would want.

The ambulance delivered Ragucci to Columbia the week after Christmas. Bad as the prognosis was, it can be hard to make long-term predictions about brain-damaged patients—at least, in the first few weeks of their condition. That meant there might be a tiny sliver of hope. Mayer told me, "When he got to Columbia, on exam he was brain-dead. His EEG was flatline. But we had no idea how much of that was irreversible brain damage and how much was the anesthesia." To get a better sense of things, Mayer wanted to take more MRI scans. But when Ragucci's mother and wife heard that Mayer was booking the imaging suite, they confronted him: no more MRIs. If the scan looked hopeless— and they suspected it would—it would take away any shred of motivation that doctors had to keep treating him.

"They said, 'We know what you're going to see. It's going to be bad. And then you're going to use it as some kind of ammunition to argue that we should withdraw care, and we're not going to do it,'" Mayer says. He shrugged and told them he would do his best.

THE REST OF the story can speak for itself—literally. My team met Ragucci six years later in an ornate, borrowed conference room at the Rusk Institute in New York City, one of the premier rehab hospitals in the country. Outside, patients shamble down the cheerfully shabby hallways, but Mark Ragucci isn't one of them. He was once, but today he's a doctor in a beige suit and a crisp white physician's coat. As a rehab specialist, he helps to restore the minds and bodies of patients facing long-term recoveries—anything from broken legs to paralyzing strokes. When he's with a patient, he talks to them constantly, guiding them earnestly and gently, even those who supposedly can't hear a thing.

Dr. Ragucci tells his story in a soft, almost apologetic voice, but I can see the same kind of stubbornness that his family showed the doctors at Columbia. By his own account, he was always that way. A wrestler in high school, Ragucci brought a wrestler's intensity to his studies at the University of Illinois, where he earned his undergraduate degree and then finished his medical degree at the College of Osteopathic Medicine. He met his wife Laura in medical school, where she was training to become a pediatrician. By the fall of 1997, they were engaged to be married and doing their respective internships at Cook County Hospital in Chicago. But then, about halfway through his training, Ragucci got a shock. He learned he had a congenital heart condition.

Ragucci has told the story often enough that he can recount it in sharp detail, as if giving a clinical presentation: "I had my first aortic dissection on January 2, 1998." He says the date with a note of defiance, maybe a remnant of the frustration of the coma patient he was, struggling to hold a thought in his head, or maybe it's just the preciseness of his medical training. In any case, the trouble started with a stabbing pain in his chest, as Ragucci was working out at the gym, fighting through a bout of insomnia between long hospital shifts.

Internship is the most demanding year that physicians will ever experience, and it was no different for Ragucci. Cook County, which in 2002 was renamed John H. Stroger, Jr. Hospital of Cook County, is iconic enough to have served as the model for television's *ER*. Large public hospitals are perfect medical training grounds, because they bring in patients with every variety of serious illness and injury, and most of the patients are poor—they have no choice but to endure the probing of medical students and new doctors. Of course, the training is well supervised. Hospitals like Cook County are elite training grounds as well as public medical facilities, and many of its senior physicians are professors at Rush Medical College.

The stress was intense. Ragucci says he regularly worked more than ninety hours a week, often staying awake nearly two days straight. As if that weren't hard enough, Ragucci had insomnia. The day his heart troubles began, he found himself sitting alone in his Oak Park apartment, after a twenty-four-hour shift followed by several hours of paperwork. "I was postcall, and I hadn't slept in about thirty-two hours. [Laura] was on call at the hospital. I couldn't sleep. So around three or four in the afternoon, I decided to go to the gym," said Ragucci.

But it was no relief. Struggling against a heavy weight, he felt a pain deep inside his chest. "I was twenty-seven years old at the time, and my first thought was, 'what the hell would I be having a heart attack for?'" recalls Ragucci. "So I waited about forty-five minutes in the locker room until the pain went away. Then I went home. I know that's probably not the smartest thing to do," said Ragucci.

"Once I got home, I called my mom—that's what you do in these kinds of situations." He paused to smile. "She said to call 911." It was January, and Chicago was digging out from a blizzard; still, Ragucci decided to walk to the hospital. He tells us he climbed over snowbanks higher than his head to reach the emergency room entrance. He found it inconceivable that he could be anything but healthy. "Going over the snow, I remember thinking, 'Hey, I'm fine,'" he said.

But inside, an EKG test was abnormal enough to alarm the attending physician. The next test, an echocardiogram, or "echo," uses ultrasound to detect abnormalities in the heart's structure. Ragucci recalls a growing sense of dread as he waited for the news—a feeling that was soon justified by the results.

"I don't really know how to read an echocardiogram, but I could see that wasn't good at all," recalls Ragucci. "My aortic valve was floppy." The aortic valve separates the left ventricle, the chamber where blood first enters the heart, from the aorta, the exit chamber. Many patients with the condition show no symptoms or just a bit of fatigue. Many live happily without ever knowing that something is amiss, but if the valve is more deformed, it can cause irregular heart rhythms or even sudden death. Ragucci's test results were so alarming, the cardiologist at Cook County recommended immediate surgery.

Ragucci is not prone to outer turmoil or emotional displays. He doesn't smile much. His curly hair is cropped short and graying at the temples, and though he looks to be in excellent physical condition, his serious aspect comes across as older than his thirty-six years. Even as he described what was probably the most frightening day of his life, his tone was flat, almost clinical.

"I think I'd just stressed my body too much," he said. Between lack of sleep, the rigors of medical training, and his insomniac gym workout, he had literally pushed himself to the brink of death. Of course, while many people keep crazy hours, Ragucci had something else working against him, genetic susceptibility. An uncle had died suddenly in his mid-thirties, presumably of heart trouble, although no autopsy was performed and the cause of death was never determined.

Fortunately, the open-heart surgery was a success, and Ragucci returned to work just six weeks later. Driven as ever, he pushed ahead with his medical training. He made no concessions to his new status as a heart patient, except for regular checkups by a cardiologist. It was nearly four years later when that cardiologist once again gave him bad news.

This time he said that scar tissue around the original valve repair was expanding, the way a garden hose starts to bulge around a tiny puncture. It could only be fixed by replacing the valve with a mechanical one. It was elective surgery technically, but as the cardiologist made clear, it was not really a choice. "They call it a semielective procedure," says Ragucci, "but what that means is that you have to do it or you're going to die."

By then, he was living in New York City, finishing his training in the specialty of rehab medicine. Though serious, the second open-heart surgery was supposed to be routine. The rate of serious complications for valve replacement surgery is only about one in fifty, and few of those complications are life threatening. Routine preoperative tests, leading up to the surgery, found nothing unusual. But there are no guarantees in medicine, and Ragucci fell on the wrong side of the odds.

"I still don't know what happened. No one does," Ragucci told me. "I figured I'd be home for the holidays." The operation was performed December 3, 2001. At first everything was routine, but then it wasn't, and all hell broke loose. Something caused Ragucci's blood pressure to drop precipitously, and the surgeons struggled to maintain the pressure. The surgery dragged on, close to twelve hours. Then Ragucci began to seize. In the recovery room, it was clear that something was wrong. The seizures steadily grew in intensity. Soon, a new one was coming every two to three minutes—status epilepticus, just like Zeyad Barazanji. An MRI scan revealed devastating injuries on both sides of Ragucci's brain.

He languished in intensive care for twenty-three days. Doctors were only able to knock out the seizures by using medication that put Ragucci into a deep coma. Each time they lowered the dose, the seizures returned. His brain was, in effect, cooking itself. By the week after Christmas, the prognosis was bleak. The family kept pressing for updates, asking if there was any sign of improvement, but after a while, the doctors could no longer hide their impatience. One exasperated physician said that they were making the ordeal more painful for themselves, looking for hope where there was none. What Laura needed to do, the doctor told her gravely, was to think seriously about taking her husband off life support. The game was over. Even if her husband's condition stabilized, the doctor said, he would be a vegetable his whole life. Another neurologist told her the same thing. There was no way her husband could recover any meaningful function. He was better off dead.

So Laura and her in-laws went looking for a second opinion. Ragucci said, "My wife called various ICUs, and someone told her there are two places you want to go. So she tried them both, and Columbia was the first place to call back."

It's the day after I've heard Ragucci tell his story, and Mayer is conducting rounds in Columbia's neurointensive care unit. A wiry bundle of nervous energy, he walks fast and talks fast, and when he and his herd of young doctors move to a new patient's room, it's hard to keep pace while simultaneously avoiding the crush of doctors, nurses, students, and visitors all pushing in the opposite direction.

Today, the nine white coats are talking about an elderly Chinese woman lying comatose in room 3, her head swathed in bandages. She was brought to Columbia after being hit by a car. Making matters worse, there were problems getting a breathing tube in, and the woman's brain was starved of oxygen for several minutes. Since arriving in the neurointensive care unit, she's had part of her skull removed to relieve the pressure, but she's been slammed with one severe infection after the other, so much that one doctor describes her as a human bacteria culture.

Mayer strides to the head of the inclined hospital bed, a dozen students and medical residents crowding in to watch. Leaning in, he begins yelling in a voice so loud that it makes the nonphysicians in the back of the crowd jump. "Li! Li!"

(To be precise, he was yelling something a bit different—we've changed the name to protect the woman's privacy.)

Gripping Li's shoulders, Mayer shakes her back and forth with a vigor that is disconcerting. Li's head flops back and forth, but her expression doesn't change, unlike the slack-jawed expressions of the medical students who look on intently. Mayer pulls up Li's eyelids and shouts her name again to no response. "No directed gaze," he mutters, almost to himself. Next, he lifts up her arm and pinches as hard as he can on two of Mrs. Li's fingernails. She grimaces slightly, and Mayer gently lays her arm back at her side.

"She's better than I remember," he says, satisfied. Mayer has seen a glimpse of life, which is all he needs to keep pushing as hard as possible. It's all relative: unresponsive as she seems, it's a tiny bit better than the day before. I could tell Mayer isn't the type of doctor to give up easily.

New York-Presbyterian Hospital/Columbia University Medical Center sits on a high bluff on the edge of the Washington Heights neighborhood. It's less than a mile from the George Washington Bridge, and on one end of the neurointensive care unit, there's a picture window overlooking the graceful towers of the bridge. From other windows you can see the chop of waves in the Hudson and the green-topped cliffs on the New Jersey side of the river. As a first-time visitor walks around the unit, there's an impression of serenity. It's like a well-run day care center at nap time. Nurses smile, doctors talk quietly among themselves.

Despite the brightness of the rooms, there's an eerie

feeling here. There's no bedside chatter, no obvious sign that until recently the men and women in these rooms were walking, talking, smiling...fathers, mothers, aunts, brothers. Almost everyone has their eyes closed, and most are hooked up to an alarming array of wires and tubes. Almost everyone looks small, surrounded by the towering machinery. Nearly all are unconscious, many with mouths agape. And that's when a darker thought strikes: this is a tomb. Many of the people we're looking at now will never make it out alive, and many of the rest will leave with their mind imprisoned in a barely working body.

In many rooms there are family members sitting at the bedside, holding a limp hand, speaking words that no one but a reporter can hear. In 2001, it was Mark Ragucci's parents in those chairs and his wife, imploring doctors to do everything and raging at the chief neurologist to not give in to his own deep doubts.

When morning rounds are over, Mayer takes a breath and talks about the patient who landed in his unit the day after Christmas in 2001. "Mark Ragucci was a case that really opened my eyes. Up to then, I mostly bought into what they tell you in the neurology textbooks, that there's nothing we can do for these patients," said Mayer.

In all likelihood, thought Mayer, he would monitor Ragucci for a few days and end up telling the family the same bad news. "I was looking at it like an act of compassion," not a medical challenge, he says. "Let's give the family some peace of mind. We'll probably end up finding the same terrible things and tell the family the same message, but at least they'll have the peace of mind to know that they went the extra mile. They tried everything."

Mayer was taken aback by the family's decision not to get another MRI, but for the next several days, his team went all out, trying to help their supposedly hopeless patient. Hypothermia has been shown to protect the brain from injury, so Mayer cooled Ragucci's body with special pads. An injured brain loses the ability to control blood pressure, resulting in dangerous swings, so Mayer's team checked the reading every few hours and adjusted Ragucci's level of blood pressure medication. Ragucci had pneumonia, so he got massive doses of antibiotics, as well. An experimental system was hooked up to continually monitor his brain for seizures that might not be evident to the naked eye.

Mayer was encouraged when the seizures didn't return, even after he had weaned Ragucci off the sedatives. Still, he showed no sign of responsiveness. Ragucci was only alive because of the breathing tube down his throat and the feeding tube implanted in his stomach. Each morning, Mayer and his residents would push, pull, and prod their patient, looking for a response. Mayer would scream out his name: "Mark! Mark!" (He generally uses a patient's first name because, he says, they're more likely to respond.)

For a long time, there was nothing. But then a funny thing happened. Something astonishing. The young physician, while still in a coma, started getting better. He grimaced when Mayer dug a fingernail into his palm. He uttered a faint grunt when Mayer shook him by the shoulders. Even as he recovered, Ragucci displayed signs of a devastating condition known as man-in-a-barrel syndrome. That is where the legs start to spontaneously move, but the midbody and arms are frozen in place. Still, it was something.

"It sounds small, but he showed small degrees of gradual improvement, from one day to the next, maybe two days later," Mayer told me. "What we've learned is that the most important sign you can see is early improvement. Even if it's as subtle as a patient starting to look over in your direction when you yell at them or reach up with a hand. Because once a patient shows you they're on a recovery trajectory, that means a healing process is in motion, and we don't know where it stops."

Within three weeks, the breathing and feeding tubes were out, and Ragucci was well enough to leave the hospital. Mayer was amazed, but he cautioned against expecting more. "I told [Mark's wife Laura], 'More likely than not, he's going to end up in a nursing home for the rest of his life. I guarantee you, he will never work again,'" Mayer said, leaning back and crossing his arms as a giant smile crept across his face. "And I was wrong."

A YEAR LATER IN late 2002, Mayer was sitting in his office when a young man walked through the door, his arms held awkwardly, his hands twisted and held rigid. It was Mark Ragucci. "I almost fell out of my chair," Mayer told me. "And the first thing he said was, 'My hands don't work.'" It was enough to nearly bring tears to Mayer's eyes.

Despite the incredible strides he had made, Ragucci was frustrated. No surprise here—any doctor will tell you that the most difficult patients are often the ones who do best. Stubborn Ragucci had an innate refusal to accept anything but total success. That's not to say he wasn't thankful. He knew he'd dodged a bullet. He confided to us that his greatest relief was being able to walk again. It's easy to see why— he's constantly moving, so much that it's unimaginable to think of him in a wheelchair.

It's hard to say how many people might benefit from aggressive treatment, like what Ragucci got at Columbia. According to the Mohonk Report, drafted by a congressionally sponsored task force of brain-injury specialists, about 35,000 Americans are in a persistent vegetative state and another 280,000 in a minimally conscious state. It's clear that many of those diagnoses are inaccurate, but at the same time, patients like Ragucci—or Terry Wallis—are still exceedingly rare.

But they happen, and when they do, they tend to make news. One remarkable example is the story of Donald Herbert, a firefighter in Buffalo, who woke up from a coma after ten years and then slipped back.[13] Dr. Nicholas Schiff had examined Herbert, and when I asked Schiff about it, he said Herbert's recovery might have been triggered by a medication he took for Parkinson's disease. A similar case involved George Melendez, a young man in Houston, who was comatose for five years after a car accident that left him underwater for ten minutes. One night, after taking an Ambien sleeping pill, he paradoxically woke up and started giving one-word answers to his mother's questions. Schiff told me that medication may have played a role in the recovery of Terry Wallis, too. About eighteen months before he began talking again, he'd been started on an antidepressant. One of his caregivers had thought he looked teary eyed, so doctors thought they'd try an SSRI.

We don't how it worked in any of these recoveries, or near recoveries, but the fact that medication may have played a role is a reminder that the amazing qualities of the mind are built on a physiological foundation. Mind *is* matter. The goal of scientists like Schiff is to understand that physiology, so that someday these patients won't require a desperately rare stroke of luck to reclaim their lives.

How do these death-defying recoveries from coma happen at all? Brain imaging technology provides a few clues, offering a glimpse of what may lie beneath the placid surface of a supposedly vegetative patient. Dr. Adrian Owen, a neuroscientist at the University of Cambridge, did an experiment with a twenty-three-year-old woman who was diagnosed as being in a vegetative state after a car accident. For five months, up to the time that Owen saw her, she remained totally unresponsive. You could poke her, shake her, and scream her name—nothing. But Owen wondered if the problem might be primarily one of communication; in other words, whether the woman might be forming thoughts but unable to tell anyone about them.

To test this idea, his team used functional magnetic resonance imaging (fMRI) to monitor the woman's brain while he played back a series of carefully spoken sentences. The fMRI detects blood flow to various regions of the brain, which serves as a marker of activity. When Owen played certain sentences, like "There was milk and sugar in his coffee," the parts of the woman's brain associated with speech comprehension lit up. By way of comparison, Owen also took fMRI readings while playing back white noise. During these interludes, the speech centers were inactive—just what you'd expect in a healthy person.

Owen also played back more complex sentences, where the meaning of a word depends on the words that follow it. For example, "The creak came from a beam in the ceiling." When he did this, the response in the speech center was even stronger. Clearly, the woman's brain was "thinking," even if she showed no outward sign of it.

And there was more. The speech fMRI findings weren't conclusive evidence of consciousness; Owen knew that people sometimes process language even while not consciously aware of it—for example, under partial anesthesia or when they're asleep. To further test the level of consciousness, Owen asked the unconscious woman to imagine playing tennis, something she had enjoyed before her accident. During the imaginary game, the fMRI detected activity in a part of the brain known as the supplementary motor area, the same activity seen in healthy volunteers actually watching a ball being bounced back and forth across the net. That cinched it. Somehow, while she was totally unable to communicate, this particular woman was not completely out of it, not at all.[14]

The most striking research, still in its infancy, involves a look at what happens to the brains of comatose patients over time. In 2006, after Terry Wallis awoke from his coma at age thirty-nine, his family allowed Schiff to peer inside Wallis' brain, using PET scans and diffusion tensor imaging. The frontal cortex, the region where most higher order thinking takes place, was full of dead areas. But remarkably, Schiff found that Wallis had grown new brain connections, working around the dead spots to connect relatively undamaged areas. There were also highly unusual brain structures developed in the rear part of the brain. When doctors scanned Wallis again, eighteen months later, the changes were even more pronounced. Schiff calls the findings "amazing."

You see, those changes are supposed to be impossible. When Schiff was getting started in neurology, he was taught that when it comes to brain injuries, "what's done is done." I was taught the same thing. Since brain cells don't regenerate when they die, it was thought that a brain injury had no chance of healing. No sensible physician would dare to cross that line in the sand, to believe otherwise, but it turns out the brain has a surprising innate ability to cheat death.

Based on a growing body of research, Schiff says that doctors need to throw out virtually everything they've been taught about the brain's ability to recuperate. To me, this relatively new field is just as exciting as the advances that might give people an extra few hours to survive a cardiac arrest. It's certainly just as meaningful—when Terry Wallis or Mark Ragucci beats the odds to awake from a devastating brain injury, it's no exaggeration to say they've been reborn.

To understand these remarkable recoveries, you have to shift your focus from individual brain cells, or neurons, to the way those neurons are organized in the brain. It still holds true that individual neurons don't regenerate that well, but what we underestimated was the extent to which a brain could rewire itself using the cells that are already there. Traditional neuroscience teaches that by the time Terry Wallis was a teenager, he had established certain pathways in his brain, allowing him to speak, think, and move. Once the brain cells were destroyed in the truck accident and by the subsequent swelling of his brain, those pathways should have been lost. Perhaps they were, but as we see—quite dramatically, in the raw evidence of the patient talking—new pathways took their place. Wallis' brain simply built a detour around the area that was damaged.

Individual neurons are much more versatile than they were once thought to be, and the same goes for specific brain regions. While neurosurgeons still throw around phrases like "the speech region" or "the visual processing region," experiments have shown that depending on the circumstances, different parts of the brain can take on the same duties. These circumstances could be carefully controlled therapy—like a stroke patient tying down his right hand to force the brain to send signals to a paralyzed left hand—or something entirely different, like the ravaged brain tissue of an accident victim like Wallis.

This phenomenon, called neuroplasticity, has been used to explain recoveries from stroke and from spinal cord injury; it forms the basis of many physical therapies, as practiced by rehab physicians like Mark Ragucci. Neuroplasticity even provides a theoretical framework for cognitive behavioral treatment in psychiatry, where patients are taught to practice helpful thoughts and behaviors and to avoid damaging or painful ones. What's remarkable about the Wallis case is that we actually have brain scans showing the new connections.[15]

"How rare is it to have a spontaneous recovery after twenty years? Rare enough to end up on the front page of the *New York Times* [which ran a story]. But for other patients to have the same capacity, we don't know the answer," Schiff told me. But, he says, no one can argue anymore that such recoveries aren't possible. "[It's] a knockdown, drag-out counterexample. And the facts of his case should make us think that it could be a lot less rare than we've thought."

Schiff is busy trying to get a large, multicenter study of coma funded and off the ground. He says, "We need to move away from just looking at what these patients can do and then looking at the calendar to see how much time has passed." To be clear, Schiff doesn't think we need to sit around waiting twenty years with every coma patient to see if they recover. Rather, he says, we should be able to develop diagnostic tools to tell us after a reasonable period of time—say, three or six months—which patients maintain the *capacity* to get better. To do that, he says, we need to figure out how consciousness really works, how neurons function together and how the brain works to mend itself.

That's a tall order. Up to now, we just haven't looked at enough patients. We know more about peering inside the brain than we did just a few years ago, but Schiff says there are many more questions to be answered: "fMRI, PET scans, EEG—all these tools are enormously important, but in isolation, individual cases don't get at the real mysterious question of what is happening in the brain during coma."

Aside from Terry Wallis, we know another person who can speak from experience. Mark Ragucci says his conscious mind was working during his hospital ordeal, even at the time when doctors and even his wife described him as vegetative, with the lowest possible score on the coma scale. It's frankly hard to comprehend. Not only was his brain badly injured by lack of oxygen, for much of that time, Ragucci lay in a medically induced coma that was meant to shut off nearly all brain activity. This is pretty remarkable. When a medical resident poked him with a small metal tool much like a dentist's pick, Ragucci didn't flinch. When his eyelids were pulled open, he didn't blink and his pupils didn't shrink. You could rub a cotton wisp across his cornea without any response. When questions were shouted in his ear, his expression didn't change. Yet Ragucci insists that the time was not a blank slate. From my perspective as a neurosurgeon, where I examine and treat patients like Ragucci all the time, what he said next was chilling.

"I remember there were voices I could hear around me. I can remember verbatim what they were saying, when I supposedly was in a deep coma at the time. I subsequently could provide descriptions of the people who were walking around my bed—and this is when I was in a pretty bad sort of way," he says. Remember, his doctors had diagnosed him as nearly brain-dead.

A handful of doctors are testing ways to speed up the growth of new brain circuits. Some are looking at stem cells to try and spark the growth of new neurons. Another promising approach is called deep brain stimulation, or DBS. Neurologists implant electrodes in the brain and connect them to a pacemaker battery in the chest. They then use electrical current to try and cajole the growth of new connections in certain parts of the brain.

For years, the leading proponent of deep brain stimulation was a doctor named Edwin Cooper.[16] I was recently shown his patent for the first DBS device back in 1975. Cooper had a few strikes against him from the start: he was a nonacademic, and he wasn't even a neurologist; he was trained as an orthopedic surgeon. For years, he struggled to get researchers to take him seriously and only recently has his theory hit the mainstream. In 2006, Schiff and Dr. Ali Rezai, a neurosurgeon at the Cleveland Clinic, reported on a man they had treated with deep brain stimulation after he had lain in a minimally conscious state for six years (he had been injured during a violent robbery). The man showed dramatic improvement. Before the treatment, he had been hooked to a feeding tube and was only intermittently aware of his surroundings. After just one session of DBS, he was able to make movements to feed himself and was able to recite sixteen words of the Pledge of Allegiance.[17] Considering where he'd been, the progress was incredible.

RAGUCCI TOLD ME, "One of the reasons I didn't do neurology is because of the fact that a neurologist will tell you what's wrong, but can't tell you what to do about it." This is conventional wisdom in teaching hospitals.

Mayer hears it all the time. "We're trying to smash that concept," he said. "What we're doing is taking the patients who up until very recently were assumed to be beyond hope, unsalvageable, and we're taking an extremely aggressive approach to resuscitating these people with severe brain injuries—hemorrhages, brain trauma, and the like."

Decades ago, modern medicine came close to perfecting the ability to keep a patient alive on the most basic level. A breathing tube and a feeding tube can keep a patient breathing—technically alive—almost indefinitely. The brain, on the other hand, was out of reach. Mayer admits readily that neither he nor anyone else truly understands what triggers the healing process in some patients, but not others. What medicine can do—neurocritical care in particular—is to provide an environment where that healing process, whatever it is, can take place.

I can tell you there's a lot of watching and waiting. Much of it wouldn't be possible without careful monitoring of the brain, something that barely existed when Mark Ragucci landed on Mayer's doorstep. "We're putting probes and monitors in that directly monitor oxygen levels in the brain," says Mayer. "We can measure the neurochemistry of the injured brain." I tell my residents, it's like rolling a video camera on the damaged brain as opposed to just getting intermittent snapshots.

At New York-Presbyterian Hospital/Columbia University Medical Center, every patient who enters the unit is hooked up to an EEG monitor to watch for seizures, and most are connected to a system that takes constant readings of oxygen. By monitoring even subtle changes inside the brain, the team is able to intervene early—for example, by giving vasopressors to raise blood pressure before it drops to a dangerous level or by giving sedatives to prevent damaging seizures that wouldn't have otherwise been spotted by the naked eye.

"When I started in this field thirteen years ago, this was really science fiction. It's like going into the black box. An analogy would be: you're fumbling around in the dark, and then all of a sudden the light goes on, and you're able to see this incredible, complex, in some ways beautiful landscape," says Mayer. "When I think back to what we used to be doing, it was like flying a plane in the dark, and you could just crash into a mountain. There could be some huge problem: a physiologic storm, seizures, or a brain injury, and we wouldn't really know until the plane crashed."

The thing is, there's no flight manual, not yet. That means neurointensivists like Mayer have to feel their way along. A good example appeared on the first day of our visit. A woman who came to the unit three days earlier has started to show an alarming pattern of brain activity. It's a slow but steady electrical rhythm known by the unwieldy name of periodic lateralized epileptiform discharges— PLEDs, for short. Less dramatic than classic seizures, they're basically invisible to the naked eye. The most you can see is a trembling of the eyelids. Without the constant monitoring, you wouldn't even know the seizures are taking place—but subtle as it is, PLEDs can be a virtual death sentence.

In any case, conventional neurology teaches that there's nothing to do for a patient with PLEDs, other than hope it goes away. But we see Mayer attempt something new—a cocktail of medications to try and drive the patient into an even deeper stupor. He'll flatten the brain waves into total silence. In three days, he'll bring her back, let the sedatives wash out of her system and see if there's improvement. Think of it sort of like rebooting her brain. "The conventional wisdom has been PLEDs aren't seizures, and trying to stop them doesn't help," Mayer said. "But we've seen the natural history enough, and it's terrible. And we're not satisfied with the status quo. I told the team, 'Let's just try this approach for now, for this particular problem, and if nobody gets better, then at least we'll know that it's not going to work and we'll come up with something else."

In this case, it didn't work, not really. A year and a half later, the patient was in a nursing home with severe disabilities—unable to speak or even feed herself. Her daughter said she doesn't regret trying "everything," but doubts she would do it again if she somehow had the chance.[18] Still, it's likely that patients do better when they have an aggressive advocate, like Mark Ragucci's family. There's clinical research to suggest that a poor prognosis does, in fact, lead to indifferent care. A 2001 paper published in the journal *Neurology* said that physicians tend to be overly pessimistic in early stroke assessment and warned that the dire assessment could become a "self-fulfilling prophecy."[19]

A much larger study was published in 2004 in the journal *Stroke*. That paper examined the fate of 8,233 hemorrhagic stroke patients in California hospitals where do not resuscitate orders, or DNRs, are commonplace and in other California hospitals where DNR orders are less common. There was a lot of variation; in some hospitals none of the patients were tagged with DNRs, while in others the rate was 70 percent. Make no mistake, even when researchers accounted for age, gender, severity of symptoms and other details, they still found that patients in the hospitals where DNRs were rare had a better survival rate.[20] They couldn't say what caused it, but it's fair to guess that hospitals that treat patients more aggressively are more likely to save their lives.

The authors of the California paper write, "Decisions to limit care are often predicated on the assumption that treating physicians are able to accurately predict outcome in the specific case at hand." Left unsaid is that those assumptions may be wrong. Joseph Fins says that aside from a few academic centers, like New York-Presbyterian Hospital/Columbia University Medical Center and his own New York-Presbyterian Hospital/Weill Cornell Medical Center, most hospitals give up on patients way too soon. "Overwhelmingly, these patients are still susceptible to undertreatment. I think this susceptibility is not so much in the first few weeks [after falling into a coma], but in the subacute and chronic phase, when there is pervasive neglect of these patients."

You might be surprised to hear that aggressive treatment is not always a good idea. One critic is Dr. Justin Zivin, vice-chairman of neuroscience at the University of

California in San Diego. He says that with patients who suffer severe strokes—or any injury due to lack of oxygen in the brain—a good neurologist can make a prognosis with near-complete certainty. Someone who has lost their most basic brain functions, says Zivin, is highly unlikely to make more than a token recovery. "The majority who recover even a degree of function still have significant deficits. Their quality of life is terrible. When you give people like that too much hope, it leads to enormous expense and bad outcomes."[21]

Mayer is unapologetic, especially when he's talking about Mark Ragucci. "All signs pointed to hopelessness and neurological futility," says Mayer. "Decisions are made every day in this country to withdraw and remove people from life support without really giving them a chance. That's really what the neurointensive care movement is all about. It's about giving people a real chance." Early in his career, Mayer was on the opposite side of the spectrum. A decade ago, he often talked about how hard it was to push families to give up—to spare themselves the torment of hope, in a hopeless case. Since then, he's made a 180 degree turn, and says it was Ragucci who tipped the scales for him.

For Ragucci, the neurointensive care unit was not a tomb, but a rest station. But was his case just a fluke? While doctors are often pressed to give odds—*What are my chances, doctor?*—the truth is that most of us hate to make predictions. Patients want certainty, but that's a lot to ask for.

Ragucci has seen the MRI pictures of his own frayed

brain. He shook his head when we brought them up. "I can't even really explain, looking at my scans, how I'm functioning," Ragucci said. And yet like anyone back from the dead, he finds it hard to imagine that it could have turned out any other way. There's an edge to his voice when he talks about his parting diagnosis from Columbia. "Frankly, Dr. Mayer's prognosis for me was very grim. One thing, and I'll always remember this, he said at one point, 'I should have listened to all the other people in my department.' He was talking about the people who were telling him not to take me on as a patient, and this was right in front of my wife."

In the first years after his return to work, Ragucci often talked with patients about his own experience. Today, he doesn't mention it unless they notice the slight unevenness of movement he still displays on his left side. He says he'd rather be seen as a doctor than as a patient now, and he's uncomfortable talking with reporters. Still, the experience shapes his own medical practice every day.

"One thing I do," he says, "especially with people who can't talk, is that I always address *them,* look *them* in the eye. I don't just start up talking to their husband or wife or whoever is with them in the room. I don't talk about 'the patient' or 'the case.'" After a pause, he looks up and starts talking again. "One thing I *am* thankful for, especially now, because I'm in the practice of reviewing charts and admitting patients, is that Stephan Mayer didn't have to take me on in the first place. He could have just said, 'This is too much to handle.'"

Mayer could have said the same to Dr. Nobl Barazangi when she called about her uncle, but he took on this case, too. Professor Barazanji looked dead to the world. Of course, Mayer was looking deeper, and for the time being, he liked what he saw. By the fall of 2006, when Zeyad Barazanji landed in the unit, there was no hesitation. No effort would be spared. The hypothermic cooling was begun. The brain monitors were hooked up. Powerful antibiotics were poured through the IV to fight back infection. A wife with red-rimmed eyes sat by the bedside hoping that her husband would once again be whole.

CHAPTER SIX

Cheating Death in the Womb

I will give you a new heart and put a new spirit within you; I will take the heart of stone out of your flesh and give you a heart of flesh.

—Ezekiel 36:26 (NKJV)

I'VE BEEN A surgeon for more than fifteen years, but I'd never seen a case like this. I was barely breathing as I watched Dr. Louise Wilkins-Haug thread a needle cautiously forward, past the bones of the rib cage. The needle snaked past the gray shadowy bone, up toward the heart. There was no patient in the room with us; Wilkins-Haug showed me the film taken during the operation. Even so, my eyes were wide and I found myself leaning closer, as I watched the point inch onward. I could imagine the concentration she must have felt, the fine sweat on her brow. She would have been talking in a gentle murmur, almost to herself, as she guided the point to its target. I was watching heart surgery, one of the miracles of modern medicine, but more amazing, the patient was not yet even born.

When we talk about high-tech interventions, fetal surgery is right at the top of the list. It forces us to ask very basic questions: Who is the patient? Can we even say that he's alive? When the first fetal surgery was performed in 1981, it shifted the line between life and death in a strange and wonderful new direction. Up until now, our story has been about cheating death, about ways to keep the clock ticking to extend the precious moments of our lives. This addresses the other side of the question: where does life begin?

With advanced medical equipment and the skills that come with repeated practice, surgeons today can fix life-threatening birth defects with a success rate that was almost unimaginable when the specialty was born in the early 1980s. To take it another step, "fix" may not be the right word. The handful of surgeons who perform fetal surgery are nipping deadly problems in the bud and preventing life-threatening conditions from arising in the first place. In doing so, they blur the definition of birth and of life itself.

The pioneer of fetal surgery in the United States is Dr. Michael Harrison, at the University of California, San Francisco, Children's Hospital. In a published reminiscence, Harrison writes that he had been nourishing "a crazy idea about fixing surgical defects before birth" ever since his first month of surgical training at Massachusetts General Hospital, in the summer of 1969.[1] "As a green and naive surgical intern, I assisted Dr. Hardy Hendren in operating on a newborn baby with congenital diaphragmatic hernia (CDH) who subsequently died." In a case of CDH, the abdominal organs are located too high in the chest, blocking the development of the lungs. Harrison wrote, "It seemed obvious to me that the baby died because the lung was too small, and the lung was too small because it was not able to grow adequately before birth, and that the only way to save the baby after birth was to fix the anatomic defect before birth."

Within days, Harrison told me, he had written a protocol for a program of animal experiments that would test this radical notion in dogs.[2] It would be nearly a decade before he could put that plan into action. In 1978, after finishing his surgical training and a stint doing research at the U.S. National Institutes of Health, Harrison found himself in San Francisco, where a small group of South African expatriates was experimenting with fetal lambs. Soon, Harrison was surgically creating birth defects in the lamb fetuses, watching to see what problems developed and then attempting surgery to correct the problem. As he learned more, he started to work with fetal monkeys; these were more challenging because, like humans, they are prone to preterm birth.

This was a fertile time for research. In weekly get-togethers, Harrison would compare notes with several other physicians who were intensely interested in repairing birth defects. Dr. Mitchell Golbus ran a clinic that scanned for and treated fetal abnormalities. Dr. Roy Filly led a group that was establishing a massive fetal ultrasound unit and tracking what happens to babies who develop problems in utero. The weekly meetings, which take place at UCSF Children's Hospital to this day, came to be what Harrison calls the "heart and soul" of the fetal treatment program.

For the first procedure in a human, Harrison zeroed in on fixing a condition called fetal hydronephrosis, where the output of urine—in a developing male fetus—is blocked. Urine backs up into the kidneys, causing potentially fatal problems, and for complex physiological reasons the fetus' lungs also won't develop. The first operation was fairly simple. Harrison took the fetus, still attached to its mother's womb, and made a tiny hole in the bladder. He inserted a catheter that could drain the urine directly into the amniotic fluid. He then placed the fetus back in the womb and sewed the incision shut. That modest effort launched a specialty that in cases like the one I saw is bearing fruit as a real, lifesaving miracle.

Fetal surgery is a desperate measure. It's generally performed only after doctors determine that the fetus would not otherwise survive long past birth. Seen in that light, the surgery is a way to cheat death. But here it gets complicated. When you talk about redefining the boundaries of life, it makes people uncomfortable. Questions about life's starting point underlie some of the most bitter debates of our time. Many modern religions teach that life begins at conception, at the moment a woman's egg is fertilized by sperm. But in the legal world, it is argued a person isn't a person until they are born. The forty weeks in between are an uneasy limbo.

As strong as emotions run around the question, in a way it's like arguing over angels on the head of a pin. No brand-new developing human could survive outside the womb at the moment of conception or for several months afterward. In the majority of cases, survival outside the womb is impossible until about twenty-four weeks of gestation, but it's equally true that intervention before that point can mean the difference between life and death. Untreated, it was clear that the heart condition of twenty-two-week-old Anders Wiley would mean almost certain doom. And there I was, watching the delicate surgery that would save his life.

None of these philosophical questions were on the mind of Anders' mother when she laughingly lay on the table for an ultrasound in an Austin, Texas, medical suite.[3] A physician herself, an ob-gyn, she was taking a turn as a patient at the practice where she worked. Known to patients by her maiden name, Dr. Grogono, Sally Wiley was pregnant with her second child. The first, a boy named Dyson, had been born just nine months earlier. When she'd gone for an initial ultrasound two weeks earlier, Wiley had been deeply anxious. At age thirty-nine, she knew full well that her child was at increased risk for birth defects, most notably Down syndrome. The test, however, put her mind at ease. Everything was normal, or so it seemed.

This time, the ultrasound was just for fun, to see how those little fingers and toes were growing. As her favorite technician swabbed cold gel across her belly, Wiley felt a surge of pleasure, thinking of the new life inside her. Now her friend could see as well, peering at the screen as the black and gray images came into focus in the darkened room. But something was wrong. The friendly cooing turned to quiet. Instinctively, Wiley raised her head toward the screen, but of course, she couldn't see the details from the table where she lay. Her friend, the ultrasound tech, was still quiet, and then said, "There's something not right about his heart."

From there, it all went pretty fast. Wiley looked at the films herself, and then she had to show them to her regular perinatologist, but it was mostly a formality. There was indeed something wrong with the tiny growing heart. A healthy heart would be symmetrical, but in this one, the entire left side was shrunken. A valve releasing blood from the heart was narrow, too narrow. As a result, there was barely a trickle of blood flowing to the left side of the heart. Without blood flow, that side of the heart couldn't grow. The condition is known as hypoplastic left heart syndrome. No one knows what causes it, whether it's genetically programmed or somehow caused by some idiosyncrasy of development. Whatever the reason, as the condition progresses, blood flow to the left side of the heart is slowly but surely choked off. A serious case is always fatal.

Wiley was in shock. "It was horrible. I had been so focused on being older and Down syndrome, I didn't even think about the other things that could go wrong. So when [my technician] said there was something wrong with the heart. . . ." Her voice trailed off.

Along with her husband Jay, a law student and former political consultant, she was faced with an excruciating dilemma. Her own doctor said there was a specialist in Boston who might be able to correct the condition, but there was no time to spare. If it weren't already Friday afternoon, he would have her on a plane already. But did she want to go? Even if surgery was successful, there could be massive complications down the road. By twenty-two weeks, the fetus relies on its own growing heart to circulate blood to the rest of the body. Wiley knew her baby's developing brain might already be injured by a shortage of oxygen. There was no way to guess the extent of the damage. Her doctor raised the possibility of an abortion, but Wiley shot that down. She and Jay had already given the baby a family name—Anderton, shortened to Anders—and he felt like part of the family.

"I've always totally supported that choice," she said, "and I always thought I'd known what I'd do, faced with the possibility of serious birth defects. But when I got the news, at twenty-two weeks, there was no question. It was already a baby. Maybe not legally, but to me."

That wasn't all. Ethical and legal concerns aside, surgery would be a risk to both mother and developing child. The conservative course would be to sit and wait. If the syndrome progressed slowly enough, the heart might still grow; if it grew enough, the defect could be corrected at birth. To go in surgically now, on the other hand, might be deadly. The slightest error, the smallest nick of the uterine lining, could trigger premature labor. If she went into labor, Wiley knew she would lose her baby.

Sally and Jay Wiley felt fortunate in at least one way: A friend whose baby had also had a congenital defect advised them to get it fixed right away. "It was such a whirlwind," Jay told me. "You're just living your life, and all of a sudden you're being told you have to hop on a plane that day. But we decided that afternoon to just go all out and do everything we could to save the baby. To just drop everything and go through with all of it." By Sunday morning, they were on a plane to Boston.

CHILDREN'S HOSPITAL IS part of a huge medical complex, a maze of buildings sprawled haphazardly across the short streets of Boston's Mission Hill neighborhood, about a mile from Fenway Park. An overhead pedestrian bridge connects it to Brigham and Women's Hospital, another huge building on the other side. At Children's Hospital, the staff will tell you pretty quickly that the first operation to fix a congenital heart defect was performed here back in 1938 by a surgeon named Robert Gross.[4] Another first took place here in 2001, when a team led by Dr. Wayne Tworetzky became the first in the United States to correct a heart defect in utero. At the time, Tworetzky called it "the science fiction procedure."[5]

Another first took place here in November 2005, almost exactly a year before the Wileys arrived. This time the desperate parents were a couple from Virginia, Jay and Angela VanDerwerken. Angela, thirty weeks pregnant, had just learned that the baby had hypoplastic left heart syndrome.

She faced a stark choice: because the pregnancy was so advanced, it would have to be open-heart surgery. Even then, doctors estimated that there was only a 20 percent chance of fixing the problem; on the other hand, the condition was so severe that leaving it alone for ten more weeks was a death sentence. Undaunted, Tworetzky, a Children's Hospital cardiologist, told the VanDerwerkens he could do it. And he did. Amazingly, the operation was a success. Grace VanDerwerken was born ten weeks later with a robust, pumping heart.[6]

Tworetzky had shared these stories over the phone with Jay and Sally Wiley and that had helped convince them to come, but he had also shared words of caution. There was maybe a 10 percent chance that Anders wouldn't survive the operation. Just a few dozen infants had had the surgery, so it was hard to know the odds. The long-term prognosis could only be a guess, just an educated guess.

The Wileys landed in Boston on Sunday afternoon. Monday morning, doctors started running a series of tests, and on Wednesday, Sally Wiley found herself lying on an operating table with Wilkins-Haug gently manipulating her abdomen, trying to gently work Anders into the proper position. Out loud, Wiley said, "I can't believe I'm here." She thought of her own patients. She had cancelled all her appointments for the week. It felt strange; she felt personally close to many patients, but right now her daily Austin work routine felt very, very far away.

Jay tried to quell the worries running through his head

while sitting in the hospital coffee shop with a friend who had driven down from Providence. He avoided saying what was really on his mind: "They told us there was a chance that the baby wouldn't even survive the procedure. There are inherent risks in any kind of invasive procedure, and if he lived, there was a chance he would still have hypoplastic left heart syndrome. If he survived the operation, they were talking about a series of future heart surgeries."

But by now there was no turning back. Getting the fetus into an accessible position can take as long as forty-five minutes, but Anders moved easily—it didn't take more than twenty minutes. As soon as he was turned in the proper direction, the anesthesiologist stepped in, and within minutes, Sally was completely knocked out. The anesthesia drugs were absorbed by Anders, too, quieting his small, jerky movements.

Wilkins-Haug worked quickly. She began by making a small incision in Sally's bulging belly. Dr. Tworetzky's description from 2002 was pretty apt. Like a lot of modern surgery, this one really looks like a science fiction movie. The only thing guiding Dr. Wilkins-Haug was the black and gray ultrasound image on a monitor, just on the other side of the operating table. As she slipped the needle through the incision, she kept an intent eye on the picture. Beside it was Dr. Carol Benson, an ultrasound specialist, who watched an identical image on a second monitor over Wilkins-Haug's shoulder. Tworetzky stood toward the back of the room. Several other nurses and technicians—about a dozen people in all—stood behind either Wilkins-Haug or Benson; among the group were two specialists in cardiac intervention who could jump in if anything went wrong with Anders' heart. They were there to try and restart the heart if it suddenly failed.

With the point of her needle just outside the uterus, Wilkins-Haug paused, cocked her head, and stared intently at the image on the monitor. Her next motion would slide the needle through the uterine wall and the chest wall of the fetus, all in one smooth motion. It would be crucial to take the proper angle. Just a few millimeters off target might puncture the wall of the heart. A bigger slip, a nick of the uterus, could send Sally into labor.

Any surgery requires precision, but this one was complicated by the fact that Wilkins-Haug would be striking at a moving target. "The baby is floating in amniotic fluid," she explains. "There's a lot more movement there than people realize." Not only was the baby gently bobbing in its fluid-filled home, there also was movement from the mother herself. Even on a ventilator, Sally's body gently rocked with the pulse of her major arteries. The movement was subtle, but keep in mind that Anders' heart, at twenty-two weeks, was just about the size of a grape. Wilkins-Haug was aiming for the left ventricle, a space no bigger than a raisin.

It is a skill that is only gained by experience. Wilkins-Haug watched her needle on a flat screen, but she was working in three-dimensional space. The fetus could roll forward or back with the motion. Over time, Wilkins-Haug has come to rely on an almost intuitive sense of touch. She says, "There's a rhythmic movement. You have to kind of find where your spot is going to be, when there won't be any countermovement rocking back towards you." Aside from the risk of puncturing something, if she bumped Anders' rib, it might be enough to jolt him out of position. That would mean halting the operation.

When she felt her needle in position, Wilkins-Haug leaned forward just a touch and felt the sharp tip slide through the uterine wall, through the surface of Anders' chest, and through the valve at the bottom of the left ventricle into his tiny heart. It had been less than five minutes since she'd made the first incision.

The needle was like a straw, and a second physician—a cardiac interventionist—threaded a small wire down the narrow channel. It was attached to a tiny balloon. The next step has been compared to fly-fishing; the wire floats in the trickling blood flow while the cardiologist waits for it to catch against the valve. When it does, the doctors inflate the balloon and stretch the opening. Right away it looked good inside Sally Wiley. On the screen, the surgical team could see a rush of blood through the chambers on the left side of the heart.

Wilkins-Haug waited about thirty minutes after removing the needle to make sure there was no bleeding and to make sure that Anders' heart didn't go into an abnormal rhythm. Everything was fine. She gave the signal, and the anesthesiologist started to nudge Sally back to consciousness. The entire procedure had taken barely an hour and a half. Now, all anyone could do was wait.

Heart surgery on someone who isn't quite a person yet is a staggering achievement, but a handful of prebirth interventions are more well established. Every year, surgeons go inside the womb to prevent major birth defects like fetal tumors, urinary blockages, and congenital diaphragmatic hernias. Each procedure is another tool to cheat death.

But as typically happens in a new field of medicine, doctors grow more comfortable with these cutting-edge techniques and look to use them more broadly. In recent years, physicians have moved to treat illnesses that are "not life threatening, but life ruining," as Michael Harrison puts it. A major trial is under way to see if prebirth surgery can prevent a crippling form of spina bifida, where the spinal cord is not fully covered, leading to lifelong incontinence and paralysis of the lower part of the body. Other procedures that are on the drawing board sound even more like science fiction. Harrison, the father of fetal surgery, talks about going into the womb to inject stem cells into the fetus, to prevent common but devastating problems like sickle-cell anemia or genetic disorders in the metabolic and immune systems. "Stem cell biology is wonderful, but the place it will pay off clinically is in the fetus," he says. "The earlier you can start a developmental change, the better it is. These diseases can be quite damaging, even by the time the baby is born."

By the time Wilkins-Haug wheeled Sally Wiley to her hospital room, the surgical team had avoided the biggest pitfalls and the operation looked like a success, but there was no way to tell, not just yet. There was still a chance that the valve could close off again. For now everyone could only sit and wait, while Anders grew inside his mother.

Wiley was in no physical pain, but the wait would be agonizing. The biggest concern was preterm birth, with the time of greatest danger being the first forty-eight hours postsurgery. At twenty-two weeks, there was no way Anders could survive outside the womb. Any birth before thirty-four weeks is considered premature, which sharply raises the chance of respiratory problems, cerebral hemorrhage, poor circulation, and a host of other problems—including a long-term risk of conditions like cerebral palsy. As you might imagine, the earlier a baby is born, the bigger the danger. Anyone born before twenty-eight weeks—when lungs reach a crucial level of maturity—faces especially daunting challenges.

Until the mid-1990s, virtually all fetal procedures were done outside the mother's body. Virtually all of these patients ended up being born prematurely. Anyone who's been around for a delivery can understand the basic problem. When the sac in which the fetus grows is torn or punctured, the amniotic fluid that surrounds and cushions the baby leaks out. Or pours out, as the case may be. When a mother's water breaks, it signals that labor is close at hand. The tearing of the sac, also called the rupturing of membranes, is more than a side effect. According to Michael Harrison, the amniotic fluid actually triggers a complex biological response, which itself induces labor. That's why a physician who wants to induce birth will simply rupture the membranes.

To do anything to the fetus surgically, there's no way to

avoid this fact of biology. You have to go through the lining of that sac. Says Harrison, "If you poke this little thin lining with a needle, you make an opening that does not heal. Fluid leaks through the hole, gets between membrane and muscle, and it's a metabolically active fluid." It turns out that even a tiny amount of that fluid is enough to cause a baby to be born several weeks before it's due. You might think it's a soluble problem, but Harrison says the human anatomy has proven trickier than expected. "We used to say, 'Oh, just make a smaller hole.' But it's a discouraging thing; we've found that using smaller instruments doesn't offer a big advantage."

A few developments have made fetal intervention far less risky, to both mother and child, than it was in the early 1990s. As we've seen already, sometimes the most important medical breakthroughs are the simplest. In the case of fetal surgery, the biggest thing making it safer and more effective was the simple ability to see the patient. The first fetal surgeries, at UCSF Children's Hospital and a handful of European hospitals, were crude. Surgeons had to open the mother's abdomen to reach the fetus. But the mid-1990s saw the development of tiny fiber-optic cameras, which could be inserted on a small instrument and send back pictures to a viewing monitor that would guide the surgeon. Michael Harrison and his colleagues at UCSF dubbed the technique Fetendo, because it reminded them of watching their kids play Nintendo video games.[7] (Dr. Hanmin Lee, the current director of fetal therapies at UCSF, smiles at the mention of Fetendo but says he prefers to talk about fetal endoscopic surgery.[8])

Another breakthrough came with the improvement of ultrasound imaging, which got to the point where the ultrasound could make out fine distinctions in a heart the size of a grape. A lot of expectant parents have watched in wonder as an ultrasound technician sends back pictures of their growing baby. This is the same technology that made possible the operation on Anders Wiley. "This is where the whole field is going," Dr. Lee told me. "We are trying to make this a minimally invasive surgery."

Making fetal intervention minimally invasive hasn't solved all the problems. Even for procedures like the one that Sally Wiley went through, the proportion of preterm births is about one in three. Preterm delivery and labor remains the Achilles' heel of fetal surgery. Says Harrison, "We've been trying for thirty years, and we've failed [to prevent preterm birth]."

For such a miraculous-seeming medical procedure, fetal surgery has seen its share of disappointments. One of the biggest involved early efforts at UCSF to repair congenital diaphragmatic hernias. CDH was one of the first problems identified as something which might be fixable in utero. Of babies born with the defect, about a third die and many more have lifelong, severe, and debilitating problems caused by stunted lung development.

Unfortunately, in the first group of UCSF patients, the babies who had surgery did even worse.[9] "We found it was probably too much of an operation," Lee says now. "It didn't really work. We just had too many problems with preterm birth and the delicacy of the fetal body at that stage."

A group of younger UCSF doctors decided to take another tack, trying a complicated procedure that involves blocking the trachea of the fetus, which causes the developing lungs to secrete fluid. They hoped that the added pressure inside the chest would push the lungs to grow. Early results were promising, but a larger study fizzled. It's not the end of the story; efforts are now under way to refine the technique, using smaller surgical tools and leaving the trachea blocked for a shorter period of time. A team in Belgium has found promising results. But even after twenty-five years of research, for a relatively simple anatomical problem, there is still no reliable fix.[10]

Of the study that didn't pan out, Lee told me, "Of course, it's disappointing that something you put a lot of work into doesn't show the benefits, but you still have a group of sick patients you have to take care of. We need to think about ways of making care better for these patients. It just makes you roll up your sleeves and say to yourself, 'You still have more work to do.'"

It's a pretty tough ledger. On one side, there are modest successes, along with a few patients stolen from the clutches of fatal illness. On the other side, there is a high risk of preterm birth, not to mention the dangers of any major operation: bleeding, infection, and complications with anesthesia—for the mother as well as the developing child. With this daunting calculus in mind, these operations are almost never done unless doctors think there is no other option—if the condition looks so debilitating that the child can't wait until he's born.

THERE ARE THOSE who say the lure of technology—the sense that "we can do it, so why not?"—has been too seductive.

One of the loudest critics, a sociologist named Monica Casper, says the biggest risk is placing too much emphasis on the health of the fetus as opposed to the mother's. In 1998, Casper wrote a book, *The Making of the Unborn Patient*, based on extensive research and interviews with participants in the UCSF fetal surgery program. In a recent article, she writes that too often, doctors ignore the fact that there's a second patient in the mix: "After all, it is only with women's consent that fetal surgery can proceed at all; it is women's bodies that surgeons must traverse to access the fetus, and it is pregnant women who assume principal risk on behalf of their fetuses. Fetal surgery is not, I argued, 'fetal surgery' at all; rather, it is more aptly maternal-fetal surgery, or just maternal surgery."[11]

Casper notes that an early logo of the UCSF program was the hand of a tiny fetus reaching out for help with no mother in sight. More importantly, she says she found a cultural disconnect between the fast-track, aggressive approach of the surgeons and the delicate emotional condition of the women who came to the center. Casper says, "I'd sit down with a surgeon, and he'd be talking about why they leave the fetus inside the woman after the procedure, and he'd say, 'The mother is the best heart-lung machine available.' "[12]

It's not that Casper thinks fetal surgery is a bad idea. "I mean, the woman *is* the best heart-lung machine available. It's just that by thinking that way, they turn her into a machine," she says. Casper thinks the risks and benefits are not always fully discussed—it's safe to say that few patients are as well informed as an ob-gyn like Sally Wiley. When the situation is a life-threatening defect—like Anders' heart condition or a total urinary blockage—the benefits are pretty clear. But the calculus started to shift with the first surgical attempts to cure spina bifida in the womb. No one would argue that curing or lessening the crippling results of that disease isn't worth some risk, but it has shifted the debate beyond the realm of cheating death.

Around the same time, a handful of surgeons reached into the womb to repair cleft palates. By intervening early, they could minimize or eliminate scarring and get a better result. Still, that meant major surgery and all the attendant risks for a condition that is not life threatening by any stretch of the imagination. For Casper, it's too much. "Clearly, anything that's cosmetic, I think it's insane to go through an intervention that could be handled postnatally."

Over the last decade since her book's publication, Casper says there's been a growing appreciation that *two* vulnerable patients are involved. Just look at the UCSF logo: today, it's a more realistic silhouette of a fetus cradled by two stylized hands. Needless to say, Casper does have critics, including Michael Harrison who calls her "a stealth radical who set out to undermine the whole process."[13] Casper's critics also include a number of antiabortion activists. She told me that after the book was published, many of these passionate activists called local radio shows to bash her and showed up to protest when she gave talks at bookstores.

From its very beginnings, it was clear that fetal surgery would become an issue in the abortion wars. A 1981 *Time* magazine article describing Harrison's first case suggested that "if fetal surgery fulfills its potential, the right-to-life argument—heretofore wielded by antiabortionists—could be used in favor of medical intervention, rather than against it."[14] More recently, research by a Vanderbilt medical ethicist, Mark Bliton, found that pregnant women who are philosophically opposed to abortion are far more likely to pursue medical intervention to save their fetus.[15]

Meanwhile, the same technology that made fetal intervention possible has been adopted—in spirit—by the antiabortion movement to try and encourage women to bring their pregnancies to term. More than a dozen states have passed laws requiring doctors who provide abortions to do an ultrasound reading on any woman who comes for an abortion.[16] Some states require doctors to show those images to the expectant mother. A spokesman for Care Net, an antiabortion group that runs 1,100 "pregnancy centers" around the country, says that 75 percent of the women who see such pictures ultimately decide not to have an abortion.[17]

Not everyone accepts that number, but there's no doubt: the visual image of a fetus, almost a miniature baby, is a powerful one. When we see a tiny image on the screen, fingers curled or reaching out, human nature tells us that's a person. Even a pragmatic surgeon feels the tug of that emotion. Before the refinement of ultrasound, Michael Harrison says, "We'd never seen inside the uterus before. We never saw the kid having troubles."[18]

Intellectually, doctors knew that birth defects developed in the womb. But it took an image to trigger the sense that something might be done about it. As Harrison observed to me, "The conceptual thing was to see that, hey, we're seeing the same problems as in babies after birth. 'Oh my gosh! You can predict there's going to be a severe malformation. Hey, you can prevent that!' And it makes sense. It's just like the early diagnosis of cancer. The sooner you catch a problem, the better the results are in treating it."

Michael Skinner, Harrison's first fetal patient to survive the surgery, is alive and well today in his mid-twenties and living in Florida. He suffered a few complications from his prebirth urinary blockage, but he has good kidney function and leads a normal life. He even came to a twenty-fifth reunion celebration of the UCSF transplant program.[19] Without the operation, there's a good chance he would have been stillborn.

When he talks about that first operation, Harrison's tone is matter-of-fact. "It was really exciting. But we'd done our homework—and we thought it was the right thing to do." By that time, the homework included more than one thousand operations on fetal lambs and nearly five hundred on fetal monkeys. "We were working like mad in the lab, and this case was just desperate enough to try it."

Harrison says the nascent fetal intervention program "was an extremely shaky and vulnerable enterprise" but adds that failures have to be expected with a brand-new, experimental surgery. It's trial and error, literally. In terms of the team's broad approach, it was crucial to choose both the right patients and the right condition to treat. Fetal hydronephrosis—the urinary blockage—was easy to detect, and as a pediatric surgeon, Harrison knew that in newborns it was relatively easy to fix. But that wasn't enough to go on. "We had to prove our thinking was correct, that if you could unobstruct the urinary tract, the kidneys and lungs *would* recover," he explains.

The team also had to figure out a way to diagnose the severity of each case. They didn't want to risk an experimental surgery on an in utero patient when the problem could just as easily be repaired in a newborn; at the same time, they didn't want to work on hopeless cases. Not only would that be a poor use of time, there were cold pragmatic reasons, too. If the surgery didn't save lives, it would be harder to find permission and funding for further research. Diagnosis was difficult, because these were patients, in the womb, whom doctors couldn't physically examine. The San Francisco group spent years developing diagnostic tricks, studying crucial markers on the sonogram and biochemical markers in the fetal urine that would signal a more severe problem.[20]

*　　*　　*

As with any potentially lifesaving procedure, there were heated discussions over when its use was appropriate. Monica Casper, who studied the proceedings of the hospital's independent review board, quotes a hospital social worker and a nurse as saying that there were cases when the medical team went ahead with surgery without waiting for approval from the hospital's internal review board. [21] In medical ethics, this is a serious violation of procedure.

In her book, the hospital is given the pseudonym Capitol Hospital, and Casper declines to say which hospital she refers to—but it seems likely that the fetal surgery program in question is the University of California, San Francisco.

Harrison insists—vigorously—that his team has always fully weighed the risks and shared the information with potential patients. Hanmin Lee says that caution continues to this day: "There was always work done first to prove it could be done safely for the mother [lab animal], and, number two, that we could successfully fix a potentially lethal anomaly. We always have to prove those things are true, before we even try it in humans."

Some programs that began with high hopes—like fetal surgery to prevent the lung problems that come with CDH—have proven disappointing. For others, the jury is still out. There is no definitive study showing that the operation performed on Anders Wiley is more likely to fix his heart condition than the traditional course of waiting until birth. When I first met the Wileys, fewer than one hundred such operations had ever been performed. Even now, the oldest survivor is just six years old. There are still major hospitals and accomplished prenatal and neonatal surgeons who do not think the benefits are proven and certainly not worth the risk to both mother and child.

After returning to Austin to organize their affairs, the Wileys flew back to Boston to wait out the final months of Sally's pregnancy. Wilkins-Haug thought she had corrected Anders Wiley's heart problem, but it would be months before anyone would know the actual outcome. It was an excruciating wait. Jay Wiley describes a miserable winter, schlepping back and forth to the hospital through the frigid Boston streets. He manages a laugh, recalling it now: "We're from Texas. We weren't used to that weather!" Sally was exhausted with the pregnancy. Jay told me, "The worst part was just being in a holding pattern week after week. We desperately wanted a better picture of his long-term prospects, but we wouldn't know that until he was born."

It was four months later that everyone got their first real look at the patient. Unlike Dyson's arrival, Jay Wiley remembers the birth of Anders as a "joyless" event. There were few smiles and many tense faces in the delivery room. It's not that he is a heartless dad; it's just that it was hard to think of this as the beginning of life, when so much work had already gone into helping this infant to cheat death.

Born a week before Valentine's Day, Anders was small, and before the day was out he faced daunting complications. "It was grim," says Jay. "I went with Anders while Sally recovered, and I could tell from the look on [the doctors'] faces and the urgency with which they moved that everyone was concerned about him not doing well." Just hours after coming into the world, Anders was rushed to the cath lab. There, cardiologists who had used a tiny balloon to stretch his heart in the womb did an almost identical procedure, inserting a small catheter to further stretch the valve inside the left side of Anders' heart.

I paid a visit the very next day, as he was being monitored in the Children's Hospital Intensive Care Unit. Any intensive care unit is a bit intimidating, with all the cold-looking, massive technology, but it's especially jarring when the patients are so tiny. The ICU at Children's Hospital is huge, full of dozens of patients at any given time. The patients, mostly newborns and preemies, are barely visible beneath the mountains of wires and machines surrounding each bed. I found Sally Wiley by Anders' bedside, squeezing his tiny hand. Right away I noticed one remarkable thing: the skin around the ribs, where the needle had passed through when Anders was just a fetus, bore no scar. But the picture-perfect exterior was misleading. Anders Wiley faced a fight for his life.

Those first weeks took a major toll. With all her medical training, Sally says she was prone to imagine the worst. "They'd tell me something, and I'd go down the pathway. If his eye looked like it drooped, I'd wonder, 'Did he have a stroke?' They'd take him off for tests, and my husband wouldn't know why, but I would know just what they were concerned about, and it terrified me."

"There was almost a shorthand between Sally and the

doctors," says Jay. "Sometimes I would come away [from a meeting with the doctor] with a good feeling about our prospects, but Sally would throw cold water on that because she could read between the lines much better than I could."

Jay was getting his own crash course in pediatric medicine. "Jay said I drove him crazy, because I was so worried about everything," Sally told me. "He wishes he'd have stayed naive."

Anders struggled mightily that first month. His breathing was so weak that doctors performed open-heart surgery when he was just three months old. It succeeded in helping his breathing, but doctors couldn't say what the surgery meant for the long-term prognosis. At six weeks, Anders was well enough to be transferred to a hospital in Austin, where he spent another six weeks before going home. Even then, he wasn't out of the woods. At eight months, Anders' heart still wasn't developing properly, and he had to be flown back to Boston for another open-heart surgery.

This time, surgeon Pedro del Nido scraped away a thick layer of cells that was partially blocking one of Anders' heart valves, causing it to stick, like a door where the frame has started to warp. This is a common complication for these tiniest of surgical heart patients. Del Nido also widened two of the valves, including the same one that had been fixed when Anders was just twenty-two weeks old.[22]

Such complications highlight the questions that still surround fetal surgery. Which problems can be headed off by early intervention, and which are unavoidable results of some underlying, unknown disorder? Did the prebirth blockage cause the abnormal tissue growth, or vice versa? "What's the chicken and what's the egg?" asks del Nido. "All we know is that the two seem to go together." The aftermath of the second surgery was painful, with repeated infections and return trips to the ICU. Slowly but surely, though, Anders crawled out of the hole. He hasn't been back to the hospital for more than a year.

That doesn't mean life is normal. Anders is on multiple medications. He's developed more slowly than the average baby and much more slowly than his big brother. Approaching his second birthday, Anders is just learning to talk and take his first steps. More distressingly, after his second bout of surgery and the ensuing complications, he lost the ability to swallow. Sally Wiley said the muscles of his stomach just stopped functioning. For a while, he had to get all his nourishment through a feeding tube. A year later, though, he was eating nearly as well as any child his age. I have to say, when I saw a snapshot of Anders in a high chair with food smeared all around his mouth, it was quite a joyful sight.

Sally Wiley says the experience has given her a whole new perspective on the problems that her patients face. "It's been a really interesting learning experience. I thought I was always empathetic to patients, but now, I get it. I get the stress," she says. "It's so much more than just having a baby in the ICU. It's every day, you have something else, something new to worry about."

After all is said and done, doctors couldn't completely cure Anders Wiley's heart defect, but it's hard to look at

CHAPTER SEVEN

What Is a Miracle?

Fragile, like the first note of a brand-new song.

—David Bailey

D R. JOHN PFENNINGER was in his kitchen on a cold, Michigan winter day. He was looking for a bite to eat when his sixteen-year-old son Matthew barged in. Dr. Pfenninger remembers it vividly. Matthew was complaining about his eyes. He said he had scratched them, putting in new contact lenses. "It's weird, Dad. I'm seeing double."[1]

You don't experience double vision from scratching your cornea, the doctor thought. Holding up an index finger, he asked, "How many fingers am I holding up?"

"Two."

"Quit clowning around."

"Two, clear as day."

That was Wednesday. On Friday, the answer was still "two." It was time to visit the ophthalmologist. They didn't know it then, as they drove to the doctor's office over the snowy midwestern roads, but they were starting a descent into hell. It was also a journey that will make you think twice about the true definition of a miracle. The story I am about to tell you is one I think of every time I walk into a patient's room as a neurosurgeon. It is a story I remember when I am about to tell a patient the worst news of all.

JOHN PFENNINGER, KNOWN to friends as Jack, was a family physician with a bustling practice in Midland. He also ran a business teaching medical procedures to other physicians and traveled the country giving motivational speeches. He had been feeling guilty about not spending time with his family—especially the two girls and Matthew sandwiched in between. Exactly one week earlier, rummaging around the basement, Pfenninger had come across a bright yellow radio-controlled airplane. It was not just any plane. This one had a story. You see, Matthew loved gadgets, loved to tinker. As a child, he was an amateur locksmith and liked to fiddle with transistors and remote control cars. He had fallen in love with the yellow plane in a catalog, and after much begging, his father agreed to split the cost. Matt put the plane together on his own. He painted it maize and blue, the colors of the University of Michigan Wolverines. But it never took off, because Dad wasn't there to help. It was one thing after another: A bit of rain. Then Dad was tired; he'd delivered a baby the night before. They needed to run errands—always something.

It was three years later that Pfenninger found the plane under a tarp in the basement. He knew Matt would still be thrilled to take it out—and he vowed to do just that, that very weekend. But it wasn't meant to be. Matt was in front of him on that cold Michigan day, and Dr. Pfenninger could tell that something was wrong.

For Matthew, things started to move fast. An MRI at a nearby clinic found a suspicious mass in his head. A second set of scans confirmed that Matt had a tumor growing at the base of his brain. There were a few days between the test and the results. Matt was sitting in class when his tenth-grade math teacher handed him a note: meet your mother by your locker. "I kind of assumed what it was," Matt told me. My heart went out to that sensitive teenager trudging past the lockers to hear what he knew must be awful, unimaginable news. In the empty hallway, underneath the fluorescent lights, he spotted his mother, her eyes already red with tears. Matt told me, "We just cried and hugged each other."

Further testing showed that Matt's tumor was a rare one, called a pineal germinoma, of which there are only about forty diagnosed in the United States each year. The family was in shock, but the news wasn't all bad: this was treatable. Dr. Pfenninger took charge, finding a national expert to treat his son. The operation would be done in New York.

First, though, there was the matter of a long-planned family vacation to Hawaii. The Pfenningers decided to go ahead with the trip, but it was impossible to ignore Matt's deteriorating condition. His double vision grew so bad that on a whale-watching trip, he couldn't make out anything beyond the boat rail.

Two days later, he was in New York City, awaiting the

surgeon's knife with the wide-eyed priorities of a book-ish teenage boy. "I wasn't scared I was gonna die, but I was pretty scared that I wasn't going to be the same," said Matthew. "I was right around the top of my class, and I was afraid I'd end up with brain damage, be disabled somehow. But I had a lot of friends praying for me back home, and I knew God wasn't going to let me die."

The Pfenningers went to a Catholic church each Sunday, and Dr. Pfenninger had briefly attended seminary school before pursuing his medical career. But theirs was not a particularly devout household. Matthew was the exception; even before getting sick, he spent time each day talking to God. "I was praying a lot," he says today. "God and I were best friends. I'd walk the dog and just be praying and talking to him and stuff, going around the block." But for the first time in his young life, Matthew was going to have his faith completely shaken.

The operation was seemingly a success—so much so that Matt's only follow-up care was radiation therapy. The radiation oncologist told him that the odds of the cancer coming back were a thousand to one. The Pfenningers' plan had worked, and they had saved their son. But it wasn't long before something strange began to happen. As the summer wore on, the normally happy-go-lucky Matt became plagued with nightmares and sank into a deep depression. Even his return to school in September couldn't shake the blues. "I was freaking out," he says. "I just wasn't myself."

In retrospect, it was a harbinger of what was to come. One day a few weeks after the start of school, Matt was scheduled for a follow-up MRI. Given the thousand to one odds, nobody was really worried. But as they stared into the radiologist's worried eyes, the Pfenningers could see immediately that something was wrong.

The new MRI showed four tumors, three in the back of Matt's skull and another at the base of his spine. Each one alone was about the size of a golf ball. The tumors were back, and the Pfenningers were devastated. Matt's mother and father went from thinking their son had been cured to feeling a paralyzing fear that they were going to lose him. Matt told me, "I still felt God was there, but I was asking him, 'You helped heal me once; why did you give it back to me?'" Matt got together with friends from the church youth group and prayed. They laid hands on Matt, and there were a lot of tears in the room. Later that night, Matt told me he saw a beautiful shooting star—a rare sight, he says, in the Michigan winter. Looking for a clue from the heavens, he took it as a good sign.

If the shooting star was a good sign, then most of the other signs were pointing the wrong way. The doctors told Matt and his family that the tumors were growing fast, frighteningly fast. Given their location, another surgery was simply not an option. Instead, his doctors ordered a course of aggressive chemotherapy. Each session was supposed to last three days, but Matt's body was overwhelmed. After the second round of chemo, he had to stay in the hospital for a full week. He was throwing up day and night and getting near-constant blood transfusions. Matt's oncologist—the cancer specialist—said his response was another bad sign;

it meant that Matt was getting sicker. As the third round of chemo grew close, Matt asked his father to try something unusual, something extremely awkward for the older man. Matt asked his father to gather everyone he knew and ask them to pray.

Pfenninger thought of himself as a man of science. Although he still went to church most Sundays, he had given up his intense religious faith more than two decades earlier. He wasn't one to pray, and public expressions of faith made him uncomfortable. But this was different—this was his son—so he agreed to do what Matt had asked. The next day, everyone who worked at the Midland clinic and many doctors at Michigan Medical Center, where Matt was scheduled for chemo, found letters in their mailboxes. "I need a favor," the letter said. "My son is dying; everything else has failed, and I need your help."

Fourteen years later, Pfenninger chokes up when he tells the story. "I just asked them to pray with me. I don't know if there's a supernatural force, but I just told them, 'Some of you are healers; we've got to be connected by more than just the mechanical things we can do.'" Matt's pastor wanted to hold the service in a church, but Jack was firm: it should be at the hospital. That was where he and his fellow doctors did their healing. That's where they would ask for help.

There is no question: the role of prayer in health and medicine is highly controversial, and yet it is an irrefutable fact that many people take the connection for granted. Walk into any church, and you'll hear prayers for the sick.

At most hospitals, chaplains are always on call. Peer around a surgical waiting room, and you will see hands clasped and voices murmuring, appealing to a higher power. According to studies, about half of all Americans say they pray to help deal with medical conditions—everything from chronic pain to cancer.[2] They pray for themselves, and even more often, they pray for loved ones. Every doctor knows patients who have asked him or her to pray for them. And many doctors also pray. I have had patients and their families bless my hands before I walked into surgery and others who have asked me to kneel down with them in the patient holding area. One family sang hymns for four hours straight, the entire length of the operation, while I removed a brain tumor from their father.

I have been a physician for sixteen years, and as a neurosurgeon, I've spent much of my life peering into a microscope, distinguishing good tissue from diseased tissue and carving out the problem with sharp instruments and electrically charged probes. I don't spend a lot of time talking about faith. I was never formally trained in the interplay between the type of healing we think of in hospitals and the type of healing that takes place in private, deep in the recesses of our own minds. Yet over time, I have come to deeply appreciate the place of prayer in the healing process.

A few years ago, this was a pretty hot research topic. There were studies showing that prayer and meditation can help your immune system and that people who are regular churchgoers tend to recover faster from serious illness. Millions of dollars were poured into further research—most notably, a study run by Harvard cardiologist Herbert Benson. The Benson-led study looked at 1,802 cardiac patients at six major hospitals. Three Christian groups were given the names of individual patients, with group members agreeing to pray for "a successful surgery with a quick, healthy recovery and no complications."

Now, you may be surprised, as I was, by the results of this study. First off, the patients who were prayed for did no better than those who received no prayers. In fact, to take it a step further, those who knew they were being prayed for actually suffered more complications.[3] Why? Well, there might be a few reasons. Some suggest that patients who are being prayed for may, in fact, be sicker than average. That reason, not the prayers, might explain why those patients did worse. It could also be that patients who knew they were being prayed for felt this extraordinary outpouring of compassion could only be warranted by a profound illness, and they adapted to fit that role. It is hard to explain, but based on my experience, no study will or should stop people from praying.

Matt Pfenninger certainly doesn't think so. He was deeply moved by what his father did. "It was a pretty ballsy thing for my dad," says Matt. "He thought he'd be laughed out of town, or maybe just his friends would show up." But when Matt and his father arrived at MidMichigan Medical Center in Midland that evening, they were floored. The auditorium, which held hundreds of people, was overflowing. The crowd was out in the hallway—doctors, friends, janitors, hospital clerks. It was anyone in the building who knew him, and a lot who didn't. It was a mixed crowd. Some were church regulars, but there was also a thoracic surgeon who told Jack, "I know there have been times when I had a patient dying in my hands, and I said a prayer, and something happened. I know it." Another doctor there, a man who had worked down the hall from Jack for ten years, told him, "I don't believe any of this nonsense, but I came here for your son." It was an extremely intense and emotional experience. By the time it broke up, Jack Pfenninger could barely drag himself home, where he collapsed in bed.

It's here where the story takes a surprising turn. Around this corner, medicine and faith came colliding together. A little flutter occurred somewhere in the universe, and the line between life and death moved once again. Just one week after the remarkable coming together of people in prayer, Matthew found himself in an MRI scanner once again. Given what had happened over the previous three months, it was a time of dread for the Pfenninger family. The remarkable prayer service was nearly forgotten and Matthew steeled himself to the seemingly inevitable.

The MRI results, though, were astonishing. The tumors were gone. Not just smaller, but gone altogether. At first, Jack Pfenninger couldn't believe that the scans he was looking at actually belonged to his son—but no, there was the shunt in Matt's head, right where the surgeon had left it to drain fluid, and there was the evidence of scarring from his previous operation. Somehow, Matt's cancer had simply disappeared. There was only one word the Pfenningers could use to describe what had just happened: miracle.

A few years ago, a similar thing happened to a man named Charles Burrows, a fifty-six-year-old Army veteran who was diagnosed with inoperable liver cancer. Two months after the diagnosis, he developed a fever and nausea and started shaking. Within days, he noticed the pain in his midsection and the obvious lump were gone. At the Phoenix Veterans Affairs Health Care System, a magnetic resonance imaging scan showed no sign of cancer. There was only "empty space" where the tumor had been, according to Dr. Nooman Gilani, who examined Burrows at the Phoenix hospital. When a befuddled Gilani did some reading to try and figure out what he'd seen, he discovered more than two dozen cases of clear spontaneous regression involving liver cancer—where the patient was completely cured, despite receiving no conventional therapy. One such patient was eighty-five years old.[4]

It's not just liver cancer. Oncologists have documented hundreds of cases where tumors, miraculously and mysteriously, simply went away.[5] In 1985, it happened to Alice Epstein, a mathematician and sociologist who was diagnosed with cancer of the kidney. Despite having the kidney removed, the cancer spread to her lungs and she was given three months to live. She decided against further surgery or chemotherapy, and yet a year later, the tumors were gone.[6]

I would be remiss if I didn't share with you what went

through my head when these stories were presented to me. Like many people trained in the sciences, I tried to come up with an explanation as to what happened. Here is one thought: What if the answer was already lying somewhere deep in our own bodies? What if their own immune system was suddenly kicked into high gear and destroyed the intruding cancer cells? A number of people whose cancers spontaneously disappeared have reported sudden illnesses like the one experienced by Charles Burrows. Perhaps the immune response launched against the infection manages to blast the tumor as well. It's certainly likely the immune system is involved somehow, and a good deal of advanced anticancer research deals with how to goad it into attacking cancer cells.

As a scientist, I am bound to try and explain these rare phenomena, as opposed to simply accepting them as divine intervention or something totally inexplicable. Having said that, as a medical journalist, I'm always on the lookout for remarkable stories. When it's a patient whose cancer spontaneously goes away or a young man whose advanced tumors disappear after a round of group prayer—well, you might call those cases miracles. But I want you to think—to reconsider—what that term really means.

This entire book is about why some people recover and thrive, even when traditional medical science and even common sense would write them off. Most doctors will tell you they don't believe in miracles. What they believe in is working hard, doing their homework, and never giving up. This is how you cheat death.

*   *   *

DR. DAVID GORSKI has a pet peeve with the term "medical miracle." Gorski is a surgeon and cancer researcher at Wayne State University, who also writes two blogs, Respectful Insolence and Science-Based Medicine. On Respectful Insolence, under the pseudonym Orac, Gorski kicked off 2008 with a New Year's resolution: "Let's not use the word miracle when we really mean 'unexpected survival.'" He says that many miracles would better be credited to first-rate medical care while others are simply the result of random chance. Calling them miracles can lead patients to miss the real story—and to pursue treatments that are ineffective or even dangerous.

Take Alcides Moreno, a New York window washer who survived a forty-seven-story fall in December 2007.[7] Sure, says Gorski, that takes a lot of luck, but it was the talent of medical professionals who saved him. "What saved the guy was the concerted effort of a lot of people. That, and all the understanding we have of human physiology," says Gorski.[8]

Gorski is a crusader for evidence-based medicine—the idea that therapies should only be used if there is solid evidence to support them. In the world of cancer, that means stomping on a lot of feel-good stories. One of his mini-obsessions was the case of Starchild Abraham Cherrix (yes, his real name), a teenager in Virginia who seemingly recovered from Hodgkin's lymphoma after a bitter legal battle over his right to refuse conventional treatment.[9] Rather than accept his doctors' recommendation of chemotherapy,

Cherrix and his family traveled to a clinic in Tijuana that offers the Hoxsey method, a sundry mixture of antimony, zinc, bloodroot, arsenic (in a miniscule dose), licorice, red clover, burdock root, Stillingia root, barberry, cascara, prickly ash bark, buckthorn bark, potassium iodide, procaine hydrochloride and vitamins, liver and cactus—as well as sulfur and talc—which is applied to the skin.[10] A court stepped in to block a return trip and forced a compromise whereby Cherrix agreed to see a local oncologist, who gave him a combination of standard radiation treatment and herbal and alternative therapies. By the fall of 2008, according to news reports, Cherrix was cancer free.

Along the way in 2007, the state of Virginia passed new legislation, Abraham's Law, giving families of children age fourteen to seventeen, facing "life-threatening disease," the right to pick—or ignore—any treatment they choose.[11] In the headlines, it was a triumph for alternative medicine. For Gorski, that's ridiculous. "There's good evidence the Hoxsey method doesn't work," he says. "It's almost certainly the radiation that shrank Abraham's tumors."

That's evidence-based medicine. Gorski rejects the concept of "healing" sites like Lourdes—where pilgrims have gone for centuries in search of divine cures—and he rejects the notion that prayer can heal, saying, "It obviously doesn't work." That pretty much sums up the point of view that most scientists take—in public. But I know it leaves a lot of them, myself included, with nagging questions. Even with chemotherapy, the speed of Matthew Pfenninger's recovery is remarkable, even astounding. Most patients would take months to show any sign of shrinking tumors, let alone making them disappear altogether. There are plenty of cases, popping up all the time, where the recovery does seem truly miraculous—at least, in the sense that a medical reporter might use it, even if a neurosurgeon wouldn't.

Sometimes it really looks like someone beat the odds, that the lottery ticket paid off. Maybe it's a miracle. Maybe prayers were answered literally, but maybe it's something else, and in these cases, it is worth digging deeper, as doctors and reporters. For one thing, you have to consider the possibility of misdiagnosis. In cases that aren't so well documented as Charles Burrows' or even Matt Pfenninger's, it's entirely possible that the person never had cancer after all. An interesting phenomenon I have seen occur in hospitals is a type of groupthink. Once a patient is labeled with a particular diagnosis or prognosis, most of the other healthcare team members tend to sign on without scrutiny. That can make a second opinion valuable, if only to lay fresh, uninfluenced eyes on the problem.

But it gets more complicated than that. The practice of medicine is always changing. There are new discoveries, and new approaches that may benefit—or harm—particular patients. On top of that, every patient is an individual unlike anyone else, in ways both known and unknown. For all the value we place on clinical trials and careful research, doctors often make judgments based on personal experience—or the experience of other doctors they know or read about. These are anecdotes, as in "anecdotal evidence." They're almost dirty words to some people—you can almost hear the sneer when they say, "There's *only* anecdotal evidence for...," but after all, each patient is an anecdote. And the reasons why some people get better while others don't are not always obvious.

Another very real possibility is that the person is just plain lucky. No one truly expects to win the lottery, but most times someone really does have the winning ticket. Here's the thing: you need to consider the statistics, the chances, the odds. When we play Powerball, we *know* the true odds. On a single ticket, it's 195,249,054 to one, if you were wondering.[12] But medicine is different. No doctor can be anywhere near that precise. We come up with estimates based on the specifics of each case, on the published research, and our own experience, but in the end it's only a guess. Perhaps a well-qualified and substantiated guess, but still a guess. The doctors who told Mark Ragucci's family to take him off life support were highly educated, well-meaning physicians with lots of experience. And they were wrong.

ON A SUMMER afternoon in 1996, a thirty-year-old man named David Bailey was hunched over the phone, his grip on the handle getting tighter with each call.[13] He was going down a list, a list he had made of people who might be able to save his life. Bailey, a highly successful salesman of computer software, was surrounded by half-packed cardboard boxes. Two weeks earlier, on July 4, he and his wife were planning to spend the holiday getting ready for a move from northern Virginia to the Boston suburbs, where he'd landed a new job. He'd driven home from Massachusetts the day before, and eleven hours in the car had left him with a splitting headache.

The morning was even worse. Packing would have to wait. Not long after breakfast, Bailey was nauseated and dizzy. He tripped and fell in the living room. "My wife called 911, and I got on the ambulance, but I thought people were just unnecessarily worried," he told me. "That's the last thing I remember."

In the ambulance, Bailey had a small seizure, and at the hospital, he had a major epileptic seizure. An MRI of his brain detected a large mass, and he was rushed into surgery that same day. He awoke four days later feeling better, until he got the news. "They told me I had six months to live," he said. "The tumor was a glioblastoma. They said, 'Good luck.'"

Of all the words you might hear in a hospital, "glioblastoma," or "GBM," may be the most chilling. Of 126 known types of brain cancer, glioblastoma is the most common, but it's also the most deadly.[14] As with any brain tumor, it is relatively rare, striking about ten thousand people a year.[15] Also called a malignant glioma, this kind of tumor tends to grow tendrils, arms growing out from the original tumor site. When I open the brain to perform surgery, I can tell you these tumors look like a little version of the monster in *Alien,* gripping its victim with these evil-looking tentacles. A malignant glioma grows fast—"highly aggressive" in medical terms. Untreated, it will double in size in just *days.* Just as dangerous, a malignant glioma is "diffuse." This means that it's made up of many different kinds of cells, which respond variously to different treatments. This is important because no single treatment can kill every kind of cell in a malignant glioma. When I talk to my colleagues in the pathology department, they remind me we don't even know how many kinds of cells there are.

Where the illness comes from is not well understood. In the vast majority of cases, the cause is a mystery, and without a known cause, doctors can't even tell you how you might prevent it. But all the research on malignant gliomas reveals an incredibly complex and resilient enemy. For one thing, cells within the tumor constantly and quickly mutate. A biopsy taken during surgery often looks dramatically different from a biopsy taken when the tumor recurs just a few months later. It's like a completely different disease. This variety of cells is referred to as heterogeneity. Heterogeneity is why doctors often prescribe multiple treatments for cancer patients; what kills one kind of cell may leave others to continue growing. Worse, an ineffective treatment leaves tumor cells that are resistant, and as they multiply, all the resulting cells will be resistant, too. A single treatment—a single chemo drug alone, for example—virtually never works.

A glioblastoma is also a physically moving target. According to Dr. Darrell Bigner, the director of the Preston Robert Tisch Brain Tumor Center at Duke Medical Center in Durham, North Carolina, its cells almost always develop the same ability to migrate through the brain, as do cells in a child's developing brain. By the time the cancer is discovered, the cells have usually crossed to the other side of the brain and sometimes down into the brain stem. For this reason, surgery is never enough to fully eliminate this type of cancer.

That's not to say surgery isn't vital to survival; in the short term, the patient needs surgery to cut away the tumor that's pressing on his or her brain. As a neurosurgeon, I've learned several techniques that make surgery an even more powerful anticancer tool than it was ten or twenty years ago. Before any operation, we create a 3-D model of the brain and the tumor, to identify precisely where the tumor is located and how that relates to the parts of the patient's brain that are critical to functions like speech and movement.

In recent years, some surgeons have learned a more dramatic way to map these vital areas. Many now perform brain surgery on patients who are not knocked out by anesthesia (this is possible because the brain itself is not sensitive to pain). Senator Ted Kennedy—who underwent surgery at Duke—was one such patient. In so-called "awake surgery," the medical team can stay in constant communication with the patient, asking him to recite a sentence or to grip a ball, in order to make sure they're not cutting into a part of the brain that would cause major damage. What this means is that surgeons can be much more aggressive; they can cut out more of the tumor, without having to leave a large margin of error to protect sensitive brain regions. But it's still not a cure. We're pretty much at a limit with what we can do surgically, because we can only take out what we can see. And at this level, the real problem is the tumor cells that we can't see.

Put it all together, and the diagnosis has been historically a death sentence. Without treatment, the average survival time is just a few months. With standard treatment—surgery to cut out the tumor, followed by radiation and chemotherapy—most patients still die in less than a year. Just 3 percent make it five years—and these are patients who are relatively young for cancer, often in their thirties, forties and fifties.[16]

A WEEK AFTER SURGERY, David Bailey went to meet with his doctor, expecting to strategize about how to save his life. "They took out the staples and stitches. And then I said, 'So what's the plan?' He suggested a guy I might want to call," says Bailey. "I said, 'Well, do you have a number?' And then, 'Can I use your phone?' I'd done some research, and I knew this thing doubled in size every ten days. Here, it had already been twelve days." Bailey could tell his doctors weren't feeling the urgency, so he had to ask, "Is this always lethal?"

"It's pretty hard to beat" was the limp reply.

GBM is such a grim diagnosis that many doctors won't even try to beat it. They'll push patients straight toward end-of-life care, treatments meant to ease suffering rather than fight the disease. But David Bailey wasn't ready for that. To find hope in a hopeless situation, Matt Pfenninger turned to prayer; Bailey turned to the Internet. He got home and started surfing the web. With an old dial-up modem, it took a while, but he found a website, www.virtualtrials. com, that listed all the experiments, all the trials of potential new ways to beat this hopeless condition. He felt a little better, but only until he started calling, with that white-knuckled grip on the phone.

"I called the first number, and said, 'Hello, I'm Dave Bailey. I have a brain tumor. Can you help?'" remembers Bailey.

"What do you have?"

"Glioblastoma."

"Ohhhhhh."

Says Bailey, "You could hear it in her voice." And in the voice of the next person he called, and the next. "I'd get that same depressed tone of voice, basically saying, 'There's not much I can do.' I'd just hang up. This was not what I was looking for."

And that's how it went, all the long, long day: one dead end after the other. But then on the twenty-fourth call, he heard something different. "This girl answered the phone, and I gave a little speech. She said, 'Oh, yeah? Tell me all about it.' Just this little change in tone. I said, 'Yeah, I'll tell you everything.' She was empathetic, caring, and at the end she said, 'I'll give the doctor all the details, and he'll call you tonight.'"

Somehow, her good-bye was a letdown; after dozens of dead ends, Bailey figured he was being blown off, again. But at ten thirty that night, the phone rang. "There was this voice, saying, 'Hi, I'm Dr. Friedman at Duke. I hear you've got a brain tumor. What are we going to do about it?' And I said, 'I don't know, but you're hired.'"

The voice on the line was Dr. Henry Friedman, the deputy director of the Preston Robert Tisch Brain Tumor Center. When I sat down and spoke with Henry Friedman, he was dressed in a Duke sweatshirt and a pair of jeans. He wasn't exactly what I expected. With almost an irreverent sense of humor, he quickly charmed everyone in the room. What struck me the most was how often his cell phone rang. I came to learn that he gives his number to all of his patients and strongly encourages them to call. It's all part of the healing that he offers.

Friedman says that what happened to Bailey is typical. "Almost every patient I see, a physician has said they're dead before they even get to us. Virtually everyone," says Friedman. Too many doctors, he says, think there's nothing to be done for patients like Bailey. That means Friedman's first battle is against perception. "You don't have to die of GBM. It's not a given, and because it's not a given, we can offer interventions that are more optimistic. Hope is the real card you play. It's very critical in any battle, against any illness." That was the message David Bailey had been waiting to hear. The next morning, he and his wife packed his brain scans into an envelope, packed up the car, and drove the four hours to Durham.

This was 1996, and after a new round of brain scans and meetings, Bailey was put on a drug called temozolomide, which today is sold under the brand name Temodar. Bailey was just the twelfth person ever to get it. Friedman was as optimistic as he could be under the circumstances. Bailey was an energetic young man, and his initial operation had cut the tumor down to the size of a lentil. And for three months, the news was good. With temozolomide, along with standard chemotherapy and radiation, Bailey's brain scans were clear.

After radiation and drug therapy, standard treatment would have been to leave well enough alone. But Bailey and Friedman weren't done. During the second surgery, surgeon Allan Friedman (no relation to Henry) had inserted a port, or shunt, a tube physically implanted in Bailey's brain through which another experimental treatment could be administered.

The approach is called monoclonal antibody therapy. Proteins from a malignant glioma are loaded onto human immune cells, which learn to react to those proteins. These cells are cloned in the lab and bonded to radioactive iodine. Administered through the shunt, the treatment is supposed to work like a smart bomb. Guided by the immune cells, the radiation goes on a search and destroy mission straight to the cancer cells, leaving the surrounding brain tissue unhurt.

For Bailey, the experience was a bit unsettling. Every day, an official from the Nuclear Regulatory Commission would come to Bailey's hospital room with a Geiger counter to make sure the radiation from the antibodies wasn't seeping into the rest of the hospital. But Bailey responded well—very well. In the vast majority of GBM cases, the cancer comes back within a few months, and the patients die a few months later. But by the time my team met David Bailey, he had gone more than a dozen years without a trace of malignant growth. That's a spectacular result. So good, you *might* call it a miracle.

But it pays to dig deeper. Scientifically speaking, Bailey is an outlier. Diagnosed with an invariably deadly brain cancer, he beat incredible odds. How? As I have said, most doctors don't believe in divine intervention; they believe that if a patient gets better, there must be a good reason. Now, we might have a tendency to give ourselves too much credit—to say that whatever the physician did is the thing that cured the patient. But there is a plus side as well. It means we are always looking for an underlying reason—a lesson to learn that might help others. It is fair to say that just because we find a scientific explanation for something doesn't make it less wonderful—less miraculous, if you will. The fact that we can detect religious feeling on brain scans doesn't make those feelings of awe any less powerful.

In any case, a survival story like Bailey's is a great big puzzle. It's a mystery where the clues are so tiny that they can only be seen at the end of a powerful microscope, in chemical bonds, and the makeup of our human DNA. It's instructive to look at the clues one by one. Think of it as the scientific dissection of a miracle. Like others in these pages who have cheated death, Bailey had a few things going for him. For one thing, he was young, and younger glioblastoma patients are known to do better.[17] Before his cancer, he was generally healthy, and he was given a multitude of treatments, some conventional and some experimental. He also got surgery, traditional chemotherapy, standard radiation, a new experimental drug, and then the experimental monoclonal antibodies. Which treatment, or treatments, was critical to his survival?

We can't say for sure. By now, many other patients at Duke and other academic cancer centers like UCLA and M. D. Anderson Cancer Center in Houston have received the same experimental treatments as Bailey did, as well as a few newer therapies. There's been a measure of success—in some studies of monoclonal antibody treatment, average survival nearly doubled to almost two years—but almost no one makes it a dozen years, certainly not without a hint of trouble.[18] So what is it about David Bailey? Is he just a statistical quirk? Does he have good luck? Did God choose to save his life? Or is there something about his story that just might help other patients?

THE PRESTON ROBERT Tisch Brain Tumor Center is a place where they try to put the puzzle together. Dr. Darrell Bigner, the director, is a soft-spoken man with a courtly southern drawl. In a storied scientific career, he has laid the groundwork for a number of cutting-edge treatments, including monoclonal antibodies, an approach that his lab first developed. Yet despite some advances against brain cancer, Bigner says bluntly that the disease is winning the battle. "It's still a poor prognosis. There have only been two new treatments in the last thirty years, and to tell you the truth, neither of them is terribly effective," says Bigner. "[On average] they might extend life, and quality of life, by just a few months."

According to the National Cancer Institute, the standard of care for glioblastoma is surgery, followed by radiation and Temodar.[19] That combination has been shown to increase average survival by about two months compared to radiation alone.[20] That's not bad, but it isn't great, either. We clearly need something better. That's why Henry Friedman and the other doctors at Duke put so much emphasis on clinical trials. About two-thirds of the brain cancer patients who come through the door at Duke are put on an experimental protocol.[21] "Surgery, radiation, Temodar—we just don't think that's good enough. We don't think that's adequate," says Friedman.

If insurers will pay—and Friedman is aggressive in pushing them—almost every patient gets something extra: an experimental drug, procedure, or vaccine, for instance. The first extra tends to be Avastin, a monoclonal antibody that works to block the growth of blood vessels that feed tumors. After years of promising results from this experimental use, in May of 2009 the Food and Drug Administration officially approved Avastin as a treatment for GBM. (It had previously been approved to treat colon cancer). Other patients at Duke are funneled toward studies on monoclonal antibodies fused with radiation—the treatment Bailey got—or to anticancer vaccines.

A Duke vaccine trial that's received a lot of attention lately involves a substance called CDX-110. In the 1990s, a number of cancer researchers—Darrell Bigner among them—noticed something unusual happening with the proteins on the cell surfaces of glioblastomas, as well as on breast, ovarian, prostate, and colorectal cancers. The protein that made them take notice is known as epidermal growth factor receptor, or EGFR. In healthy cells, it binds to another protein, epidermal growth factor (EGF), part of a process that's vital to the controlled division of cells.

The researchers noticed that there was a lot more EGFR

on the surfaces of tumor cells than there was on the healthy cells. What's more, cancerous cells often display a mutation of EGFR, a version with a name right out of a *Star Trek* episode: EGFRvIII, or EGFR factor three. According to Dr. John Sampson, a cancer specialist at Duke, if EGFR is a switch controlling cell division, EGFRvIII is a switch that's "on" all the time—constantly signaling the tumor cells to divide.[22]

Identifying this protein meant that cancer specialists had a target. Scientists from several major centers, including Duke, Stanford, Johns Hopkins, and M. D. Anderson all played a big role. They took a portion of the EGFRvIII protein and combined it with other substances that send the body's immune system into overdrive. When injected, the vaccine triggers the body's immune system to attack any cell that's loaded with the mutant version of EGFR—in other words, the tumor cells. It's like a heat-seeking missile. In an initial study where patients got CDX-110 along with Temodar and radiation, the vaccine more than doubled survival time. The average patient lived more than two years, instead of just a year.[23]

At Duke, the difference is palpable. Patients used to go home for a few months and die—now they come in with complaints like broken bones from skiing accidents. Says Sampson, "We see people back now that are having complaints and problems that you just don't *see* in people with brain tumors. Like a guy four years out [from his diagnosis], who should have been dead three years ago—he's out skiing, and hurt his knee."

Imagine hearing stories like this when you've just been given six months to live. They mean hope. Sampson says, "You can't give people hope, unless you can show people someone who's done well. It's like jumping out an airplane without a parachute. You can be as optimistic as you want on the way down—it doesn't change the outcome. But it's different if you can point to a second rip cord."

Now, the CDX-110 vaccine is being tested in a larger study, at twenty cancer centers around the country. As high as hopes have risen, we need to remind ourselves that the therapy is largely unproven. But CDX-110 is part of a larger trend toward personalized treatments for cancer. Because it targets the mutant EGFRvIII protein, it only works against cancers that express the protein—about 40 percent of all glioblastomas, according to Sampson. At Duke, genetic screening is now the norm. At Duke and other centers taking part in the current trial, tissue from every malignant glioma is tested to see if it contains EGFRvIII. If it does, these patients get an EGFR inhibitor as part of their treatment. This is complicated stuff and full of uncertainty, but this is how miracles are made and how their mysteries are unraveled as well.

As the patient, you want to try everything; you don't want to leave any stone unturned. As the doctor, you know you have to weigh potential benefits against the risks, since side effects can literally be deadly. But most researchers— though of course many are doctors, too—have a different mind-set, and this brings up another problem. They're trying to zero in on the right treatment—to solve the puzzle—and if you throw the kitchen sink at a patient, you can't isolate what works and what doesn't.

To be clear, most major cancer centers do offer multiple treatments for patients. But the holy grail of cancer treatment is a way to predict which approach will help which patient. Here, genetic screening may help. Of more than twenty thousand genes that lay the foundation of our bodies, researchers have already identified about twenty that seem to be related to the incidence of brain tumors. With that information, they've identified a few specific genes that seem to signal whether a particular treatment will work in the first place before the treatment is ever given. Temodar, for example, only seems to help about 30 percent of glioblastoma patients, those who carry one particular gene.[24]

Even as a surgeon, I can tell you that the future of treatment will lie outside the operating room. Remember, this is still a disease with no cure. I think the future for David Bailey and countless others around the world does involve personalized medicine, keeping in mind that glioblastoma is different in various groups of patients. It is true that all these tumors look the same when you're staring down at them in the operating room, but when you look under a microscope and break them down on a molecular or genetic level, it's different. One day we'll have more examples like Temodar—we'll know that if you have x gene, you'll respond to y treatment. I also suspect that, someday, genetic profiling will explain those extremely rare cases, like Chuck Burrows or Alice Epstein, whose bodies are able to somehow reject cancer on their own. It will be further proof of something we have known all along, that every patient is different—and that every tumor is different as well.

FOR DAVID BAILEY, a diagnosis of deadly cancer was a new beginning—not the end. About six months into his recovery, his hair still gone from radiation therapy, Bailey was sitting in his Virginia living room, waiting to see if the monoclonal antibodies would keep the cancer at bay. By then he'd gotten to wondering about what he should do with his life, whatever was left of it. The job in Massachusetts was gone. Between the headaches, surging emotions and memory problems, selling software again seemed unthinkable. As he sat on his couch, sunk in thought, Bailey's wife placed a guitar in his hands. He had plucked away during high school and college but hadn't touched the instrument in years.

"I started crying," he remembers. "I had lost some vision, and I didn't even know if my fingers worked. But I started going, started playing again that same day. It just unlocked a whole bunch of things." He started practicing and writing songs. With each passing week, he gained strength in his hands. With each MRI that came back clean, he gained confidence, and before long, he was performing in local coffee shops. In two years, he had his first CD—of more than twenty.[25]

Along the way, he's played in forty-four states and

Europe, in every sort of venue, but he says he finds the gigs for cancer groups especially meaningful. "I step back and remember," says Bailey. "For a lot of people in the audience, me just stepping on stage and saying, 'Twelve years [since his diagnosis]' is the victory."

He told me, "I remember in those first weeks [after the diagnosis], I went for this long walk, and on this walk I did what I assume a lot of people do. I got pissed off at God, waved my fist at the sky, and I cursed, 'Why me?! Why me?!' And I tell that story, and the audience always understands. These days, I imagine God saying, 'Wrong question. Don't ask 'why?' Ask, 'What now?' It's a huge epiphany. But it adds a huge responsibility. You realize you're not the total victim you maybe thought you were."

Here's how he put it in a new song "Fragile."

Lookin' in from the outside
Don't know what to say
Storms will come every day
But even hurricanes go away
You just learn what it takes to be strong
Don't have to be fragile very long

To beat stupendous odds, to make a miraculous recovery, you need a few crucial ingredients. You need a patient with the inner strength not to give up and the wherewithal to seek help. And you need a doctor who is willing to try almost *anything*. You need hope—the kind of hope that Henry Friedman offers. The kind of hope that guides him in making a million tiny decisions, medical calls, and trial and error that add up to lifesaving treatment.

"The motto is so simple," says Bailey. "'At Duke there is Hope.' But it's amazing: so many people miss the boat about how important that is. For us, there is no such thing as false hope. There's hope, and there's no hope. I weave this into my concerts, telling people, you've got a choice: dig in your heels, wrap yourself around hope, or crawl into a corner and die. There's nothing in between."

DARRELL BIGNER BROUGHT up something I had wondered about when I first learned of David Bailey's story. Until the 1990s, he told me, pretty much every long-term glioblastoma survivor was probably a case of misdiagnosis: some other, less aggressive tumor. In Bailey's case, that's not the issue. Multiple brain scans and biopsies at a top-notch cancer center left no doubt that he had a deadly glioblastoma. At the time he was first diagnosed, there was no one, literally no one, who could say they'd survived the illness for more than a decade. And yet in 2008, we found him alive and well, just like the title of his latest CD.

Bigner says there are more stories like this one to come. "We don't want patients to think this is a hopeless situation. Unfortunately, unless you are actively trying to cheat death, this is what we're told by the vast majority of the medical profession. Our patients hear it all the time: 'You've got this malignant brain tumor; there's nothing to be done but palliative care. Go write your will, take a nice vacation and get ready to die.' And that's not really the case at all."

When Henry Friedman criticizes other doctors for giving up on their patients, he uses the same words as Stephan Mayer and Lance Becker: "therapeutic nihilism." That's the notion that nothing can be done. For some terminal patients, that's true. But even with an illness as deadly as glioblastoma, there's hope if you're willing to take a fresh look. "The status quo is unacceptable," says Friedman. "If we use the same interventions we've always used in the past, there's no reason to think the outcomes will be any different, but if we are hopeful and use interventions that are new...." his voice trails off for a moment. "Well, then the canvas is totally unpainted."

It certainly echoes the stories we've heard about other patients left for dead. Back in 1996, when David Bailey was diagnosed with brain cancer, a skier like Anna Bagenholm, who was trapped under freezing water for two hours, probably never would have made it to a hospital. A cardiac arrest victim like Zeyad Barazanji—who had stopped breathing for five minutes—might have been left to languish in a coma. Not to mention Mark Ragucci, whose doctors said was doomed to life as a vegetable, if he lived at all. Like other doctors we've met in these pages—Stephan Mayer, Gordon Ewy, Mads Gilbert—Friedman isn't waiting until he has all the answers. He works with what he has, pushing his patients—and colleagues—to try something new. The more they try, the more patients who decide to fight, the more David Baileys we're likely to see.

MATT PFENNINGER'S STORY is a little different. Pineal germinoma—Matt's brain tumor—is not invariably fatal.

Overall, the survival rate is around 60 percent, according to the American Cancer Society. Still, to beat cancer is almost always a long and winding path, and that brings us back to the Pfenninger home in Midland.

You see, just six months after the deeply moving prayer service and Matthew's miraculous recovery—well, that's when the story really begins. The tumors came back. In fact they recurred in two places on either side of his brain. The locations were so delicate that surgery to remove either tumor was out of the question. "That was the beginning of the worst part," Matt told me.

At that point, the Pfenningers, like so many others before them, made their way to Durham, to the Preston Robert Tisch Brain Tumor Center and Dr. Henry Friedman. Under the care of Friedman and a pediatric oncologist, Dr. Joanne Kurtzberg, Matt underwent a series of bone marrow transplants. His condition improved enough for him to fulfill a lifelong dream by attending the University of Michigan in Ann Arbor. But it wasn't meant to be. A few weeks into his freshman year, he dropped out. Matt told me, "I could barely eat anything. There was a hole starting to form in the roof of my mouth as a side effect of all the medications. It was not fun. It's supposed to be the best time of your life, and I couldn't have been more miserable."

What Matt went through the next two years is frankly too horrible to imagine for most people, but he recounted it for me with astonishing detail. There was surgery to remove a tumor that had spread to his lung. An artery and a vein became fused, which led to another surgery, taking out a third of the lung. Another day, sitting down to a meal of tacos at home with his father, Matt felt liquid in the back of his throat. Standing over the sink, he coughed up two liters of blood. He made it to the hospital, choking blood into a salad bowl while his father drove. He passed out in the waiting room. "I felt like I was going to die," he told me. "It was pretty peaceful. I was sad for the people I was leaving behind, but I wasn't scared at all." The nurses desperately packed his nose full of cotton to stop the bleeding.

From there it was back to Duke, for another bone marrow transplant. On this go-round, Matt jokes that the only doctor he didn't see was the gynecologist. The family ran up $2 million in medical bills, as Matt got daily blood transfusions for three months. He had a throat full of tumors, with constant blood clots that threatened to cut off his breathing. One day he passed out from loss of blood and had an emergency tracheotomy. He ended up on a respirator. He couldn't eat; five months into his hospital stay, he had a tube in his gallbladder and a feeding tube in his stomach. The first time medical staff put in the feeding tube, it wasn't tightened properly and it leaked, so he ended up with a severe infection inside his abdomen. He could no longer go to the restroom on his own.

Throughout the seven-month hospital stay, Matt's mother, grandmother, and sisters took turns by his bedside, while his father kept up the home in Midland. More than once, Jack Pfenninger got a call from Duke, telling him to get down there, that his son might not make it through the night. At that point, says Matt, "I was just waiting to die. I was ready to go. The doctors kept telling me it was going to be okay, but I was pretty convinced it was over."

One especially painful day, Pfenninger leaned across his son's bedrail and whispered the most difficult words he'd ever spoken: "If you want to let go, just let go. I won't hold you. I'm not going to make you suffer." After hugging his son, Jack had his hand on the door to leave, when Matt managed to speak, saying, "Dad, I love you. And I want to come home." Jack took it as a stubborn promise.

No one knows what makes for a turning point in a long illness like the one that almost killed Matt Pfenninger. But right around the day of that promise, his condition took a turn for the better. Maybe that's as much of a miracle as the time his tumors went away after the round of group prayer. In any case, the next MRI showed the tumors in his brain were stable. The next thing he knew, they were shrinking. Less than two months after his dad's visit, Matt staggered off a plane in Midland, looking up at a skywriter's message: "Welcome Home, Matt." It was Father's Day 1997.

The scars are still there, figuratively and literally. To remove one of the tumors, doctors had to cut out part of Matt's vocal cords. His voice is raspy and so high it almost squeaks. But somehow, after three years doing battle with cancer, Matt picked up at almost the same place he left off. He returned to college, graduating from Saginaw Valley State University, near his home, with close to a 4.0 grade point average. Then he made it back to Ann Arbor, where he picked up a degree in electrical engineering. Today he designs software for General Electric and marvels at what was almost his fate.

Whether or not you believe in divine intervention, even some hard-core scientists and cancer specialists see real value in positive thinking, which Matthew almost always maintained. On the most basic level, research tells us that a positive attitude goes along with a stronger immune system; one study even found that people who meditated or prayed were more resistant to a flu virus that was blown into their noses. Beyond that, I believe strongly that the will to live is real. This may just be that a person who decides to fight his disease is more aggressive in seeking care. Any doctor will tell you that the most difficult, complaining patients are usually the ones who do best. Think of Mark Ragucci. Or it may be that someone healthy enough to fight is just more physically resilient.

Many people lump all this together as "the biology of hope." David Gorski, the skeptic, isn't sold. "I don't reject it out of hand, but I don't think the current state of research supports it." On the other hand, Dr. Henry Friedman—as serious a scientist as there is—says there is no question: hope is a lifesaver. Even if he's not sure how it works.

Friedman told me, "I think the real message is that if you enter with a philosophy that cancer patients will die— well, then they die. But if you go all out to help them, an ever-increasing number survive."

A skeptic would say that the prayers for and by Matthew Pfenninger didn't really work. After all, the tumors came back again and again. If he got better, it's because he had state-of-the-art treatment at Duke. But even in that select group of patients, quite a few don't make it. We'll never know why Matt was one of the lucky ones. His faith is stronger than ever, but at the same time, the illness left him with a sense of unease, as if the ground beneath him had shifted. He struggles to put the feeling into words, then tells me, "I haven't figured it all out yet. It's been years and years, and I haven't figured out what it meant to my life. But I think there's a lot more to God and to Jesus than meets the eye."

Jack Pfenninger says there are still times he finds himself consumed with what was lost. "I'm still so angry about it. I ask Matt, 'What do your friends think of all those scars?' You had to give up the Fulbright scholarship—you lost your youth—aren't you angry?' And he tells me, 'No, I'm the luckiest guy in the world. I walk and talk, I feed myself, I play music [Matt is an amateur guitarist and songwriter], and I'm an engineer. If you weren't a doctor and hadn't noticed the problem with my eyes, I'd be dead.'" To this, Jack Pfenninger adds, "I'm a scientist. I don't understand why he was healed. He should have been dead. Who saved him? God? I don't know."

Whether we're a doctor or a patient, we tend to think that life and death are somehow under our control, and to an extent, they are. That's why we go to the doctor in the first place, to help us heal. That's what motivates doctors like Henry Friedman and the other medical mavericks we've seen in these pages. They push the boundaries of our

CHAPTER EIGHT

Another Day

Lateat scintillula forsan. (A small spark may perhaps lie concealed.)

—motto of the Royal Humane Society

W HEN WE LEFT Zeyad Barazanji, he was lying in a medically induced coma. He had survived a cardiac arrest, nearly four minutes of clinical death, and a hairline fracture in his skull, but he was still deep in the woods. Doctors at New York-Presbyterian Hospital/Columbia University Medical Center had cooled his entire body with special pads to try and minimize the swelling and inflammation. The procedure typically takes about three days—then you wait. But here it was, a week later, and the pads were back on. This time the goal was to cool the fevers that were boiling Barazanji's system.

He couldn't feel a thing. The usually nimble brain, the mind of a professional translator who could understand four languages, was utterly quiet. To quell the constant seizures that rippled through Barazanji's brain and kept it from healing, the doctors put their patient on heavy doses of powerful sedatives. They had driven him into what's known as a medically induced coma. All they could do was wait. He had arrived November 7. Now, it was November 18.[1]

It was hardest on Raoua Barazanji. Born in Syria, like her husband, she had met him in the Bronx fourteen years before and married him a few months later—on New Year's Day in 1992. She was his second wife, and they had no children, though Zeyad had a grown daughter from his previous marriage. He was everything to Raoua. By day and most nights, she kept a vigil by the bedside, her gaze shifting from the sunlight pouring through the windows to the mass of tubes and wires that were propping up her husband, figuratively and maybe even literally. When she left these days, it was home to the Bronx, where she spent most of her time calling relatives with updates. She tried to keep up her spirits by cooking some of Zeyad's favorite Syrian dishes.

She would go to bed, the smells of dinner still hovering in the air, then wake and ride the subway across the bridge to Manhattan to her husband's side. The mornings were usually easier, surrounded by friends, some from as far away as Damascus. When Raoua was alone, the frustration could be too much. She would find herself standing over the bed, shouting, "Wake up! Open your eyes!" Sometimes he would open his eyes. The first time he did, Dr. Mayer, the head of the neurointensive care unit, was surprised. But he said it happens that way sometimes. They would keep their fingers crossed. Raoua would tell herself that she could see

Zeyad's chin jutting out, the way it did when he was feeling stubborn. He couldn't move, but he was sending out a message: I'm not going anywhere.

On the nineteenth of November, friends and family were putting on their coats and getting ready to leave Zeyad's bedside. They asked Raoua where they might try to grab a bite to eat downtown, when there came a voice from the bed. Something about "the Village." Raoua and the two friends turned and stared. The voice was coming from underneath all those wires; it really was. The words didn't quite make sense, but there was her husband, awake, playing the gracious host. There were a few bumps after that—another fever, a bad case of shingles—but twenty days later, Barazanji was out of the hospital. He looked like a skeleton. He'd lost more than 65 pounds off his 185-pound frame. But he was alive. He had cheated death.

There's no simple answer as to why Zeyad Barazanji cheated death when so many others who suffer cardiac arrests don't make it. The truth is, *most* don't make it. But, Barazanji had been fortunate in many ways. There was that quick response of bystanders and paramedics and the help from his niece who steered him to state-of-the-art treatment. Dr. Stephan Mayer, who puts so much faith in therapeutic hypothermia and the growing specialty of neurointensive care, thinks cooling was a crucial component. An unavoidable comparison was the young man in the room literally next to Barazanji. He had arrived the same day, but only after lingering nearly three weeks in another hospital, without being cooled. He died just a few days after

Barazanji walked out of the hospital.[2] There but for the grace of God...

Barazanji's friends like to joke about his stubbornness. Barazanji told me, "I don't remember it, but my wife says I pulled aside one of the doctors or nurses and told them, 'Listen, I am not an easy patient. I am too demanding.'" As you may have gathered, I do believe there's something tangible about the will to live, a certain inner strength. Whatever it was, something stopped the hourglass before it ran out. Barazanji was dying—he was clinically dead—but then the clock was reset.

IN THIS AND other cases, the line in the sand is shifting, reflecting the excitement of new technology and also the uncertainty that comes with it. I once thought death was inalterable, but Dr. Lance Becker, the director of the Center for Resuscitation Science at the University of Pennsylvania School of Medicine, says medical advances have changed its very definition. "The language of death will always contain one of two words that should bother everyone," says Becker. "'Irreversible' or 'permanent.' That's kind of funny, because if you think about it, 'irreversible' and 'permanent' are only words you can use in retrospect."

If you ask Mark Roth, the scientist who's been putting animals into suspended animation, whether death has taken place, he'll say something similar. "I don't know. How long did you wait?"

This might sound like pointless wordplay, but it has

a direct impact on clinical practice, on the care of real patients. Becker estimates that he's pronounced about a thousand people dead over the course of his twenty-five-year medical career. Like other doctors, he has to fumble along the best he can. According to Becker, here's how it usually happens at the Center for Resuscitation Science: "You're working, doing everything you can. The guy doesn't have a pulse. You don't have another drug. You sit there, and say to one of the residents, 'Okay, hand me the chart; let me see if something else is going on.' You read the chart. Then you start asking people on the team: 'Can you think of anything else to do? Can you?' And when no one else has any ideas, we call it." Time of death, 2:15 a.m.

Can you really define death as the moment that doctors quit? "Yes, that's what I believe," says Becker. You can say to yourself that he must be exaggerating, that doctors don't really argue about death like that—but as my team did research for this book, we ran across all sorts of examples where the line in the sand was not clear at all.

Some of them are pretty bizarre. We heard about a case in Haiti, involving a man named Clairvius Narcisse, who died in a Port-au-Prince hospital in 1962 of what his doctors described as malnutrition.[3] He—or at least someone—was buried in the local cemetery. But in 1980, a sick, elderly man appeared in Narcisse's village claiming to be Narcisse. His sister and several other family members immediately recognized him. What happened in the eighteen years in between remains unclear, but Narcisse and his family claim he was drugged and kept as a slave on a distant sugar plantation. He said he escaped after the plantation's owner died and the poison wore off.

Chalk it up to the curse of the zombie. In Haitian folklore, a witch doctor can gain control of a victim's mind with black magic and keep him or her in a state between life and death—as an undead. Far-fetched as it may seem, a Canadian ethnobotanist and anthropologist named Wade Davis claims to have found some real evidence—not of black magic, but of something equally strange. In the 1980s, Davis spent time in Haiti, where he befriended voodoo priests who gave him—he claims—a "zombie powder," which he tested in a Washington, D.C., laboratory. (He later detailed the experience in two books, *The Serpent and the Rainbow* and *Passage of Darkness*.) According to Davis, the powder's key ingredient was tetrodotoxin, the same substance found in the lethal puffer fish. The victim ingesting the powder would be immobilized with a near-lethal dose; as it began to wear off, the zombie would be aware of his or her surroundings yet unable to move. Supposedly, victims like Clairvius Narcisse could then be enslaved for years, kept in a fog or trance with drugs like scolopamine, atropine, and hyoscyamine, the chemicals found in hallucinogenic plants like Datura or nightshade. The zombies look dead, were pronounced dead, and yet are here are among the living.

The details of Davis' work are controversial,[4] but there's a natural fascination with stories like these, and it often shows up in popular culture—and not just in horror movies about zombies and the undead. Back in the early nine-teenth century, catalogs and fashionable stores sold an array of coffins equipped with features such as air hoses, glass lids, and ropes that could be tied to bells at the graveyard surface. The most famous "bell" coffin was known as the Bateson Life Revival Device. From today's vantage point, it looks like paranoia, but the craze stemmed from a new medical advance: the emergence of rudimentary mouth-to-mouth resuscitation and defibrillation techniques. Then, as now, the public was fascinated by a handful of tales about patients literally brought back from the dead. I should point out that there is no documented case of one of these "safety coffins" actually being put to good use, but there *are* documented cases right here in the modern United States, of patients who were taken to the morgue and put in the freezer before they woke up and started calling for help.[5]

AS FASCINATING AS I find these stories, the true scientific advances of people like Mark Roth and Lance Becker are something I find even more exciting. They remind us that for all the progress we've made, we've still only scratched the surface when it comes to cheating death. Some branches of medicine are able to manipulate death so easily, it barely raises an eyebrow. At the Center for Resuscitation Science alone, twenty to thirty patients have their hearts intention-ally stopped each day, when they have an internal defibril-lator implanted. It only lasts a few seconds, but those few seconds are indistinguishable from the first few seconds of a cardiac arrest like the one that almost killed Zeyad

Barazanji. As long as the clock has barely started ticking, it's no big deal to bring you back from the dead.

"At time zero, survival is fabulous," Becker says. "It's pretty good up to five minutes. But if we could extend that window to thirty minutes, it would save 200,000 people a year." From seconds to minutes to hours and days, with interventions like therapeutic hypothermia and possibly hydrogen sulfide. How far can it go? At Alcor, the cryogenics foundation, they've had nearly a thousand customers willing to pay $150,000 apiece to have themselves put into a deep freeze, to await some as-of-yet-unknown medical miracle. They're betting their inheritance that by the time they're unfrozen, doctors will know how to fix any damage that the process may have caused.

The military is pushing hard to find better methods of trauma care, and by extension, ways to extend the clock. Another frontier, as they say, is outer space. If we humans ever get around to traveling beyond our solar system, we'll need an effective means of suspended animation. Otherwise, even traveling at the speed of light, any astronaut would die long before reaching his destination.

There are special challenges when it comes to this realm of research. We're talking about life and death, not good skin care—the stakes could not be higher. Especially in the United States, this makes it difficult to obtain approval for major studies, where a new treatment is tested against a control group that gets the standard treatment or even no treatment at all. Ethics councils and review boards play an important function, helping patients avoid unnecessary risks, but there also are risks to sticking with the status quo. Look at what happened with therapeutic hypothermia. Despite its immense promise, the treatment ran into a catch-22—one government agency said there wasn't enough evidence to approve its use, but no one could get more evidence because another agency said it was already obvious that the treatment works and that it would be unethical to withhold it.[6]

Research on emergency care can provide critical insight by challenging conventional wisdom. Here's one example: Since the 1970s, it's been standard of care to treat cardiac arrest by giving a shot of epinephrine—adrenaline—along with any CPR and defibrillation. But doctors in Norway just finished a study that lasted five years, with more than a thousand patients, comparing the survival of patients who received epinephrine during their cardiac arrest with patients who did not. There was no difference in survival.[7] The standard treatment didn't help at all.

A few months before those results were announced, a popular television reporter, an investigative journalist named Tarjei Leer-Salvesen, got wind of the study and did an expose. He called the study a "lottery," where lifesaving treatment was withheld from half the patients.[8] There was such an uproar the study was cut short.

You can see the problem. When we challenge conventional wisdom, we may find that treatments we've taken for granted—like traditional CPR—aren't terribly effective, and we may find newer approaches that work better. In the example from Norway, it turns out the lifesaving treatment, epinephrine, wasn't really lifesaving at all, and if the study had been cut off sooner, no one ever would have known. Dr. Kjetil Sunde, one of the authors, was still furious when my team met him a few months later. He told us, "People only think you're a good practitioner if you give a lot of drugs. If you just cure him with traditional doctor's wisdom, they think you're bad."

In fact, what I've seen again and again while writing this book is that simple treatment can indeed be the best lifesaving method when it comes to emergency care. Therapeutic hypothermia is decidedly low tech. You can produce the effect using bags of ice. The biggest breakthrough in emergency resuscitation of the past thirty years is a new version of CPR that involves nothing more than pressing the victim's chest firmly and rapidly.

Speed and simplicity are a mantra for Dr. Mads Gilbert, the daring physician who saved Anna Bagenholm from the frozen stream where she spent two hours underwater. Gilbert spends a lot of his time as far away as you can get from the frozen fjords of Norway. He makes several trips a year to developing countries, bringing basic supplies to strapped physicians (as in Gaza) or teaching basic emergency medical techniques to laypeople in places that are out of the reach of emergency medical technicians.[9]

Gilbert helped develop this emergency curriculum, which is called the Village University. It's already made a big impact. One of Gilbert's first projects was in northern Iraq; another was in Cambodia, where forty-year-old landmines take a tremendous toll in the rural countryside. In these two far-apart regions, the fatality rate from landmine injuries fell from 40 percent to just 15 percent, after two intensive training sessions of twelve to fifteen days each, under Gilbert's direction.[10] There was no medical breakthrough, no high-tech drug for the battlefield. Gilbert and his colleagues simply taught the farmers and village leaders how to properly stabilize a wound and helped them develop transportation networks—mostly by motorbike—to speed the delivery of victims to formal medical care.

He's set up similar village universities in Burma and Angola with similar success. Gilbert says, "It's the simple things, not the sophisticated things. We saved all these lives just by working with what you'd call barefoot doctors, training in basic techniques that are usually reserved for academic doctors, at least in our part of the world."

It's a lesson being learned here as well. In the field of emergency care, Lance Becker says the biggest change on the horizon is a breaking of walls between traditional specialties. To use therapeutic hypothermia on a patient isn't technically complicated, but it takes a lot of coordination. Everyone from the emergency room staff to the cardiology team to surgeons to neurointensive specialists all need to be on board. That's a problem, says Becker. "Right now, we have an organ mentality. There's been this two hundred–year period, where cardiologists take care of the heart, and pulmonologists handle the lungs, and kidneys are for the nephrologists, and on and on. It's like the blind man looking at various parts of the elephant."

We now know that death is a complicated thing. Actual

death doesn't happen in just one organ at a time. It's almost always a system-wide breakdown, a cascade of unfortunate events, unfolding inside every cell. "We need an integrated systems approach," says Becker. "And I predict we'll see that change within ten years. I'm hopeful, because there's a coming together of a lot of this science. There will be some unifying kinds of therapies. But we're not there yet."

The psychologist and author Robert Kastenbaum has written quite a bit about the concept that death doesn't happen in a moment but rather unfolds over time. At any point, it just might be stopped, it just might be cheated. Although it may be cutting-edge science, Kastenbaum says it harkens back to older beliefs:

> Historical tradition . . . has often conceived death as a process that takes some time and is subject to irregularities. This process view has characterized belief systems throughout much of the world and remains influential in the twenty-first century. Islamic doctrine, for example, holds that death is the separation of the soul from the body, and that death is not complete as long as the spirit continues to reside in any part of the body.[11]

None of the exciting medical changes that we've come across will ever give us total control over death. They won't eliminate the sense of awe and mystery that stalks our notions of death. And I have a feeling they will never answer some of the nagging questions that confront every patient with a life-threatening illness or the doctors who care for them.

When a patient is lying close to death—Mark Ragucci, for instance—the family hopes for a miracle. But what, exactly, does that mean? In the sometimes faceless, technologically driven world of advanced medicine, doctors tend to be uncomfortable about discussing just how much uncertainty remains in what they do. Doctors are said to "practice." The implication is they don't quite have it down. And it's true.

What makes for a miracle can only be understood through the filter of our current knowledge and our own expectations and hopes. One of the most remarkable people we came across while writing this book was David Bailey, the software salesman turned musician, who fought off a deadly brain tumor with the help of experimental treatments at the Preston Robert Tisch Brain Tumor Center. He was given six months to live. When my team first met him, it had been twelve years cancer free. But the week we were finishing the first draft of the book, we got this e-mail:

"...Don't know if you heard, but long story short I spent the last week at Duke for a semi-emergency brain surgery (#3) to remove an 8cm fluid filled cyst and an odd tumor that is now being biopsied.

Home now, feeling much better. getting used to the train track on the side of my face. :-) Let me know if there's anything I can do—and have a great thanksgiving.—lots to be thankful for(!)

David

The cancer was back. That wasn't how the story was supposed to go. It doesn't make it any less of a miracle that Bailey lived twelve cancer-free years with an illness that kills most people in a few months. But it's still a gut punch for all the doctors he has encountered and the friends that Bailey has made on his incredible journey. At the time of this writing, he was back at Duke for another round of monoclonal antibody therapy—the same experimental treatment that saved him all those years ago, now refined, we hope, to be even better.

When someone dies of illness, we say they died of natural causes. But it's just as natural that we fight it. We cling to life like a drowning man clings to a life raft. Life is the only thing we know.

In Zeyad Barazanji's living room, we could see the sun getting low, as the hum of conversation grew louder in the living room and mouthwatering smells wafted out from the kitchen. Barazanji gestured to the door and said he wanted to show us something. We walked down the stairs, a spring in his sixty-eight-year-old steps, out the back door and onto the sidewalk. We strolled in the warm late summer afternoon, a block down the steep winding hill, tracing the edge of a park where dog lovers walked and the voices of children rang out on a playground. Barazanji pointed out what he said was the oldest building in Riverdale, and from there it was another half block along the promenade, overlooking Henry Hudson Park. We stopped at the top of the next staircase, broken stone steps leading down into the park. This was his favorite spot, he said, where he walked during his rehab, where he came when he wanted to watch the trains heading up to Connecticut, the boats on the Hudson, the sunset beyond. He closed his eyes. Death was nowhere to be seen.

Notes

PROLOGUE

1. The story of Zeyad Barazanji is based on interviews with the author and his team, and on this article: "Return of the Ice Age: Therapeutic Hypothermia in Emergency and Critical Care," *P&S* (in-house journal for the College of Physicians & Surgeons of Columbia University) vol. 27, no. 3 (Fall 2007).

CHAPTER ONE: ICE DOCTORS

1. Unless otherwise noted, information on the Anna Bagenholm case comes from three sources: interviews conducted by the author and his team with Mads Gilbert and Anna Bagenholm; and "Resuscitation from accidental hypothermia of 13.7°C with circulatory arrest" by Mads Gilbert and others, from *The Lancet* 355, no. 9201 (2000): 375–76.
2. The cases of Mandy Evans and Canadian toddler Erika Nordby were widely described in contemporary news reports.
3. The experiments of Walt Lillehei and the University of Minnesota produced historically important scientific research that was vital in the development of cardiac surgery, transplant surgery, and other specialties. A gripping account for lay readers is included in Donald McRae's book *Every Second Counts.*

4. L. P. Kammersgaard and others, "Admission body temperature predicts long-term mortality after acute stroke," *Stroke* 33 (July 2002): 1759.

5. Matt Andrews, PhD, of the University of Minnesota, in interview with the author's team. Another source of wisdom on ground squirrels is Hannah Carey, PhD, of the University of Wisconsin.

6. For a few days, Gilbert was a favorite target of conservative websites in the United States and Great Britain. Two examples can be seen at http://confederateyankee.mu.nu/archives/280821.php and http://www.hurryupharry.org/2009/01/07/mads-gilbert-doctor-pundit-shill-for-terrorism/. As an interesting side note, CNN was criticized for showing video of Gilbert in a Palestinian hospital, assisting with CPR on a boy in a manner that several critics described as fake. CNN pulled the video from circulation to give me a chance to observe it and assess the veracity of the resuscitation effort. To me it was clear that the effort was real, though futile, in that the badly wounded patient was beyond the point of no return.

7. All accounts of earlier efforts at the University Hospital of North Norway to resuscitate severely hypothermic patients are based primarily on the recollections of Dr. Mads Gilbert.

8. Dr. Nobl Barazangi is the daughter of Zeyad's brother, who spells the family name differently.

9. Several psychiatrists confirmed that cold sheets were widely used in psychiatric hospitals in the first part of the twentieth century. Dr. Julie Holland of NYU suggested another reason they may have been effective; she pointed out research by Temple Grandin, PhD, showing that simply being held tightly can have a calming effect, in particular lowering the respiratory rate. Being wrapped tightly would presumably

do the same. The cold—depressing temperature and metabolism—would magnify the effect.

10. Stephan Mayer in interview with the author's team.

11. I covered Richardson's death for CNN. Her injury, known as an epidural hematoma, is generally fatal unless surgery is performed within a few hours of the injury.

12. Donald W. Benson, "The use of hypothermia after cardiac arrest," *Anesthesia & Analgesia* 38, no. 6 (1959): 423–28.

13. Suad A. Niazi and F. John Lewis, "Profound hypothermia in man," *Annals of Surgery* 147, no. 2 (February 1958): 264–66.

14. Benson, "Hypothermia after cardiac arrest."

15. Mayer, interview.

16. Stefan Schwab et al, "Feasibility and Safety of Moderate Hypothermia After Massive Hemispheric Infarction," *Stroke* 32, no. 6 (June 2009): 2033–2035

17. Andrea Zeiner et al, "Mild resuscitative hypothermia to improve neurological outcome after cardiac arrest: a clinical feasibility trial," *Stroke* 31, no. 1 (January 2000): 86–94.

18. "Mild therapeutic hypothermia to improve the neurologic outcome after cardiac arrest," *The New England Journal of Medicine* 346, no. 8 (February 2002): 549–56.

19. "2005 American Heart Association guidelines for cardiopulmonary resuscitation and emergency cardiovascular care," *Circulation* 112, no. 24 (December 2005): IV-136–IV-138.

20. U.S. Food and Drug Administration, Center for Devices and Radiological Health, Circulatory System Devices Panel, minutes of meeting on September 21, 2004.

21. U.S. FDA, CDRH, minutes from meeting on September 21, 2004.

22. Carmelo Graffagnino, MD, Duke University, in interview with the author's team.

23. Edna Kaplan, Medivance spokeswoman, in interview with author's team.

24. Marcus Ong and others, "Controlled therapeutic hypothermia post-cardiac arrest compared to standard intensive care unit therapy," presentation to the 2006 Society for Academic Emergency Medicine.

25. Raina M. Merchant and others, "Therapeutic hypothermia utilization among physicians after resuscitation from cardiac arrest," *Critical Care Medicine* 34, no. 7 (July 2006): 1935–1940.

26. Raina Merchant in interview with the author and his team.

27. http://www.med.upenn.edu/resuscitation/hypothermia/protocols.shtml

28. Zeyad Barazanji's medical records.

29. Mary Grace Savage in interview with the author. Her husband, Patrick Savage, is a deputy chief with the FDNY; a detailed timeline of his rescue was laid out in the *New York Daily News* on July 3, 2007.

30. John Freese in interview with the author's team.

31. I came to know the work of Audrey de Grey while researching my previous book, *Chasing Life*. Among other things, I had dinner at the home of his research assistant, Michael Rae, who is practicing another radical longevity strategy: a diet of severe calorie restriction.

32. Jennifer Chapman in interview with author's team.

33. CBS's *The Early Show*, February 3, 2000.

CHAPTER TWO: A HEART-STOPPING MOMENT

1. Unless otherwise noted, information on the Mike Mertz case comes from interviews conducted by the author's team with Mike Mertz, Corey Ash, and Chuck Montgomery, Glendale Fire Chief.

2. Bentley J. Bobrow, "Minimally interrupted cardiac resuscitation by emergency medical services for out-of-hospital

cardiac arrest," *Journal of the American Medical Association* 299, no. 10 (March 2008): 1158–1165.

3. Benjamin S. Abella, "Reducing barriers for implementation of bystander-initiated cardiopulmonary resuscitation," AHA Scientific Statement, *Circulation,* published online January 14, 2008.

4. U.S. Department of Health & Human Services, Agency for Healthcare Research and Quality, http://www.innovations .ahrq.gov/content.aspx?id=1737.

5. Gordon Ewy in interview with the author's team.

6. Myron L. Weisfeldt and Lance B. Becker, "Resuscitation after cardiac arrest: a 3-phase time-sensitive model," *Journal of the American Medical Association* 288, no. 23 (December 2002): 3035–3038.

7. Ewy, interview.

8. American Heart Association, "About sudden death and cardiac arrest," http://www.americanheart.org/presenter.jhtml ?identifier=604.

9. Leonard Cobb et al, "Influence of cardiopulmonary resuscitation prior to defibrillation in patients with out-of-hospital ventricular fibrillation," *Journal of the American Medical Association* 281, no. 13 (April 1999); 1182–1188.

10. Gordon A. Ewy, "Cardiocerebral resuscitation: the new cardiopulmonary resuscitation," *Circulation* 111, no. 16 (April 2005): 2134–2142.

11. Gordon A. Ewy, "Continuous-chest-compression cardiopulmonary resuscitation for cardiac arrest," *Circulation* 116, no. 25 (December 2007): 2894–2896.

12. Ewy, interview.

13. Mike Kellum in interview with the author's team.

14. Mercy Health System website, http://www.mercyhealth system.org/body.cfm?id=7

15. Kellum, interview.

16. M. Kellum, K. Kennedy, and G. Ewy, "Cardiocerebral resuscitation improves survival of patients with out-of-hospital cardiac arrest," *The American Journal of Medicine* 119, no. 4 (2006): 335–340.

17. Mike Kellum and others, "Cardiocerebral resuscitation improves neurologically intact survival of patients with out-of-hospital cardiac arrest," *Annals of Emergency Medicine* 52, no. 3 (September 2008): 244–252.

18. Bentley Bobrow in interview with the author's team.

19. We spent time with several paramedics in Glendale during the writing of this book; all recalled intense initial skepticism about Bobrow's approach. Perhaps the most interesting story came from paramedic Crystal Sorenson. A day before he visited her firehouse, she had performed a highly unusual resuscitation on a dog belonging to her son's girlfriend. The dog had apparently collapsed with no heartbeat, due to an allergic reaction to a bee sting. While Sorenson dug through the house for a shot of epinephrine, her son, on her instructions, pressed on the dog's chest, but—as you might imagine—gave no rescue breaths. Despite more than ten minutes with his heart stopped, after receiving the shot of epinephrine, the dog revived with no obvious long-lasting ill effects. With that experience fresh in her mind when Bobrow gave his presentation, Sorenson was more receptive than most to the new protocol.

20. Bobrow, "Minimally interrupted cardiac resuscitation."

21. Taku Iwami, "Effectiveness of bystander-initiated cardiac-only resuscitation for patients with out-of-hospital cardiac arrest," *Circulation* 116, no. 25 (December 2007): 2900–2907.

22. I found another simple but successful intervention in an unlikely spot. Perhaps no public place on earth is so closely watched as the gaming floor of a Las Vegas casino. Secu-

rity cameras hang in every conceivable location. In the mid-1990s, Dr. Terence Valenzuela of the University of Arizona realized that the cameras—and the people watching them—could do more than scan for drunks, card cheats and criminals. Valenzuela and colleagues convinced thirty-two casinos to install automated defibrillators in all public areas, trained the security guards to use them, and taught them basic CPR. Over the next two and a half years, 105 casino patrons suffered what doctors would consider a "survivable" cardiac arrest. More than half the victims lived to walk out of the hospital, at least ten times better than the typical survival rate. To this day, the safest place to have your heart give out is probably the floor of a Las Vegas casino. (As detailed in *The New England Journal of Medicine* 343, no. 17 (2000): 1206–1209.)

23. R. Dunne and others, "Outcomes from out-of-hospital cardiac arrest in Detroit," *Resuscitation* 72, no. 1 (2007): 59–65.

24. Graham Nichol and others, "Regional variation in out-of-hospital cardiac arrest incidence and outcome," *Journal of the American Medical Association* 300, no. 12 (September 2008): 1423–1431.

25. Graham Nichol, director of emergency care at the University of Washington Harborview Center for prehospital care in Seattle, in interview with the author's team.

CHAPTER THREE: SUSPEND DISBELIEF

1. This estimate is based on the following: the LC-50 (concentration that would kill half the people exposed to it) for hydrogen sulfide is 800 parts per million. That can be converted to 0.8 grams per liter. Fanciful as it may be, one could thus say that 0.8 grams of H_2S could kill approximately half the people exposed to it; therefore an ounce of H_2S could

kill approximately 18 people. This experiment will not be conducted any time soon.

2. This is based on standard material data safety sheets; these are two examples: www.mathesongas.com/pdfs/msds/MAT11210.pdf and http://avogadro.chem.iastate.edu/MSDS/hydrogen_sulfide.pdf

3. Mark Roth in interview with the author.

4. Roth was named a 2007 Fellow by the John D. and Catherine T. MacArthur Foundation.

5. Brett Giroir, former DARPA director, and Jon Mogford, director of DARPA's Surviving Blood Loss Program, in interviews with the author's team.

6. In 2007, Ikaria merged with a more established biotech company, New Jersey–based INO Therapeutics, which had existing facilities for the production of gas-based medical therapies. Several news reports put the value of the merged company, Ikaria Holdings, at $670 million. The company has approximately 300 employees.

7. Many news outlets, including CNN, covered Uchikoshi's hospital news conference on December 20, 2006. That remains the only time he has spoken of the incident in public.

8. The precise triggers of apoptosis remain a subject of intense research, but the role of cytochrome c has been detailed by several scientists. The primary source for this description is an interview I conducted with Dr. Lance Becker of the Center for Resuscitation Science.

9. Roth, interview.

10. Roth, interview.

11. Roth, interview; Pamela A. Padilla and Mark B. Roth, "Oxygen deprivation causes suspended animation in the zebrafish embryo," *Proceedings of the National Academy of Sciences* 98, no. 13 (March 2001): 7331–7335.

12. Roth, interview. The television documentary was "The Mysterious Life of Caves," on *Nova*.

13. Some scientists believe that our cells naturally produce minute quantities of hydrogen sulfide, and that our ability to use the molecule may be an artifact of prehistoric evolution, when certain microbes used it as a nutrient, in the absence of oxygen. See Katharine Sanderson, "Emissions Control," *Nature* 459 (May 2009): 500–502.

14. Roth, interview.

15. Eric Blackstone, Mike Morrison, and Mark B. Roth, "H_2S induces a suspended animation–like state in mice," *Science* 308, no.5721 (April 2005): 518.

16. Atul Gawande, "Casualties of war: Military care for the wounded from Iraq and Afghanistan," *New England Journal of Medicine* 351, no. 24 (2004): 2471–2475.

17. Giroir, interview.

18. Michael Morrison and others, "Surviving blood loss using hydrogen sulfide," *Journal of Trauma-Injury Infection & Critical Care* 65, no. 1 (2008): 183–188.

19. Neel R. Sodha and others, "The effects of therapeutic sulfide on myocardial apoptosis in response to ischemia-reperfusion injury," *European Journal of Cardiothoracic Surgery* 33 (May 2008): 906–913; Florian Simon and others, "Hemodynamic and metabolic effects of hydrogen sulfide during porcine ischemia/reperfusion injury," *Shock* 30, no. 4 (2008): 359–364.

20. Ralf Rosskamp, MD, Ikaria Vice President of Research and Development, in interview with author's team.

21. National Institutes of Health website. The updated status for Ikaria trials can be found by visiting www.clinicaltrials.gov and searching for Ikaria. http://www.clinicaltrials.gov/ct2/results?term=ikaria

22. David Lefer in interview with the author.
23. "Severe heart attack damage limited by hydrogen sulfide, study shows," *ScienceDaily*. Retrieved April 17, 2009, from www.sciencedaily.com/releases/2007/09/070919093319.htm.
24. Lefer, interview.
25. Matt Andrews in interview with the author's team.
26. Kathrin Dausmann and others, "Physiology: Hibernation in a tropical primate," *Nature* 429 (June 24, 2004): 825–826.
27. Jeff Williams, CEO of VitalMedix, in interview with author's team.
28. Andrews, interview.
29. A signature paper of Chaudry's appeared in the *Archives of General Surgery*, vol. 138 in 2003 (pages 727–734). An overview of his work can be seen by running a PubMed search: http://www.ncbi.nlm.nih.gov/sites/entrez?cmd=Search&db=pubmed&term=Chaudry%20IH
30. Irshad Chaudry in interview with the author.
31. A CNN crew interviewed Dr. Alam and filmed one of his swine surgeries for a story that aired November 10, 2006.
32. National Center for Injury Prevention and Control, WISQARS Leading Cause of Death Reports, 1999–2005: http://webappa.cdc.gov/sasweb/ncipc/leadcaus10.html.
33. Philip Bickler in interview with the author.
34. Roth, interview.
35. I explored the science of survival at high altitude in the 2004 CNN documentary *Life Beyond Limits*.

CHAPTER FOUR: BEYOND DEATH

1. The description of Duane Dupre's heart attack, near-death experience, and subsequent resuscitation is based on his own account, given in an interview with the author's team.

2. International Association for Near-Death Studies website, http://www.iands.org.
3. Raymond Moody, *Life After Life* (Harrisburg, PA: Stackpole Books, 1976).
4. Sam Parnia in interview with the author.
5. Parnia, interview; Desmond Smith's case is described more fully in Parnia's book *What Happens When We Die?* (Carlsbad, CA: Hay House, 2006).
6. Parnia, *What Happens When We Die?*
7. Parnia, *What Happens When We Die?*
8. Bruce Greyson and others, "Failure to elicit near-death experiences in induced cardiac arrest," *Journal of Near-Death Studies* 25, no. 2 (2006): 85–98.
9. Jean Potter, a woman we met through an Atlanta group affiliated with the International Association for Near-Death Studies, in an interview with the author's team.
10. Dirk de Ridder and others, "Visualizing out-of-body-experience in the brain," *The New England Journal of Medicine* 357, no. 18 (2007): 1829–1833.
11. Strassman has written extensively about this theory, most completely in his book *DMT: The Spirit Molecule* (Rochester, VT: Park Street Press, 2000).
12. Andrew Newberg and Eugene D'Aquili, *Why God Won't Go Away* (New York: Ballantine Books, 2001).
13. Kevin Nelson in interview with the author's team.
14. Moody, *Life After Life* (2001 ed.), 16.
15. The author explored this subject in detail for CNN's 2006 documentary *Sleep*.
16. Kenneth Parks was acquitted of murder on May 26, 1988. The case was widely covered at the time.
17. Anahad O'Connor, "The Claim: Blind People Do Not See Images in Their Dreams," *New York Times,* December 15, 2008.
18. Kevin Nelson and others, "Does the arousal system contribute

to near-death experience?" *Neurology* 266, no. 66 (2006): 1003–1009.

19. In addition to medical science at high altitude, the authors explored extreme cold-water swimming for CNN's 2004 *Life Beyond Limits* documentary.

20. Jeffrey Long and Janice Miner Holden, "Does the Arousal System Contribute to Near-Death and Out-of-Body Experiences? A Summary and Response," available at http://www.nderf.org/longholdenremintrusion.pdf.

21. Jeffrey Long in interview with the author's team.

22. Pim van Lommel and others, "Near-death experience in survivors of cardiac arrest: a prospective study in the Netherlands," *Lancet* 358, no. 9298 (2001): 2039–2045.

23. Pim van Lommel in interview with the author's team.

24. Pim van Lommel, "About the Continuity of Our Consciousness," available on the website of the International Association for Near-Death Studies, http://www.iands.org/research/important_studies.

25. Michael Sabom, *Light and Death* (Grand Rapids, MI: Zondervan, 1998).

26. http://www.myspace.com/pamreynoldslive. Along with a personal account of her NDE, the website includes music tracks from *Side Effects of Dying*, a 2005 CD she released as half of the duo Reynolds Robinson.

27. Nelson, "Does the Arousal System Contribute to Near-Death Experience?"

28. Susan Clancy, *Abducted: How People Come to Believe They Were Kidnapped by Aliens* (Boston: Harvard University Press, 2005).

29. Larry Squire in interview with the author's team.

30. Post-traumatic stress and other intense memories were examined in the 2005 CNN documentary *Memory*.

31. CNN's *Memory*.

32. Pamela Wedding in interview with the author's team.
33. Nelson, interview.
34. William Kuchler, a near-death experiencer who was introduced to me by Dr. Sam Parnia, in interview with author's team.
35. Van Lommel, "Near-death experience."
36. Van Lommel, interview; Van Lommel, "About the Continuity of Our Consciousness."
37. Van Lommel, "About the Continuity of Our Consciousness."
38. The so-called AWARE study (Awareness during Resuscitation) was announced at a United Nations symposium, September 11, 2008.

CHAPTER FIVE: WHAT LIES BENEATH

1. Unless otherwise noted, the information on Mark Ragucci's case came from the following: interviews by the author and his team with Dr. Stephan Mayer and Dr. Mark Ragucci; "Against All Odds," *NYU Physician* (NYU in-house magazine), Summer 2008; and Thomas M. Burton, "In a Stroke Patient, Doctor Sees Power of Brain to Recover," *Wall Street Journal*, November 23, 2005.
2. We chose not to identify the hospital where Mark Ragucci was initially treated, due to the sensitive nature of his story.
3. Donald McRae, *Every Second Counts* (New York: Putnam, 2006).
4. McRae, *Every Second Counts*.
5. *The Mohonk Report* (2006)
6. Joseph Fins in interview with the author's team.
7. Jerome Groopman, "Silent Minds," *The New Yorker,* October 15, 2007.
8. Groopman, "Silent Minds"; "Man Speaks After 19-Year Silence," CNN.com, July 8, 2003.

9. Nicholas Schiff in interview with the author's team; Henning U. Voss, "Possible axonal regrowth in late recovery from the minimally conscious state," *Journal of Clinical Investigation* 116, no. 7 (July 2006): 2005–2011.

10. Fins, interview; Schiff, interview.

11. Unless otherwise noted, the information on Zeyad Barazanji's case comes from the following: interviews with Stephan Mayer and Zeyad Barazanji, and Barazanji's medical records.

12. A note on names: As is common in Syria, Raoua has officially kept her maiden name, Sadat. However, she frequently uses the last name Barazanji; and that is what I've used, for the ease of the reader.

13. Anderson Cooper, "Awakening," *60 Minutes*, November 25, 2007.

14. Matthew H. Davis and others, "Dissociating speech perception and comprehension at reduced levels of awareness," *Proceedings of the National Academy of Sciences* 104 (2007): 16032–16037.

15. Voss, "Possible axonal regrowth."

16. Gary Greenberg, "Back From the Dead," *Wired*, September 2006.

17. N.D. Schiff, "Behavioral improvements with thalamic stimulation after severe brain injury," *Nature* 448 (2007): 600–603.

18. Mayer, interview.

19. K.J. Becker and others, "Withdrawal of support in intracerebral hemorrhage may lead to self-fulfilling prophecies," *Neurology* 56 (2001): 766–772.

20. Claude Hemphill III and others, "Hospital usage of early do-not-resuscitate orders and outcome after intracerebral hemorrhage," *Stroke* 35 (2004): 1130–1134.

21. Justin Zivin in interview with the author's team.

CHAPTER SIX: CHEATING DEATH IN THE WOMB

1. Michael Harrison, "The University of California at San Francisco Fetal Treatment Center: a personal perspective," *Fetal Diagnosis and Therapy* 19, no. 6 (2004): 513–24

2. Unless otherwise noted, descriptions of the early fetal surgery program at the University of California at San Francisco are based on interviews with Michael Harrison by the author and his team.

3. I first reported portions of Anders' story on the CBS *Evening News*, February 28, 2007. Unless otherwise noted, the story told here is based on interviews with the following people: Sally (Grogono) Wiley, Jay Wiley, and Dr. Louise Wilkins-Haug.

4. Children's Hospital website, http://web1.tch.harvard.edu/clinicalservices/Site457/mainpageS457P5sublevel6.html

5. Denise Grady, "Operation on Fetus's Heart Valve Called a 'Science-Fiction Success,'" *New York Times*, February 25, 2002.

6. Scott Allen, "A Medical First Helps Baby Girl Beat Odds," *Boston Globe*, January 28, 2006.

7. Michael Harrison, "Personal Perspective," *Fetal Diagnosis and Therapy*.

8. Hanmin Lee in interview with the author's team.

9. Michael Harrison, "A Randomized Trial of Fetal Endoscopic Tracheal Occlusion for Severe Fetal Congenital Diaphragmatic Hernia," *New England Journal of Medicine* 349, no. 20 (2003): 1916–1924.

10. Lee, interview.

11. Monica J. Casper, "Fetal Surgery Then and Now," *Conscience*, September 22, 2007.

12. Monica Casper in interview with the author's team.

13. Michael Harrison in correspondence with the author.

14. "Surgery in the Womb," *Time*, August 10, 1981.

15. Mark J. Bliton, "Parental hope confronting scientific uncertainty: a test of ethics in maternal-fetal surgery for spina bifida," *Clinical Obstetrics and Gynecology* 48, no. 3 (2005): 595–607.

16. Associated Press, "Kansas Governor Signs Abortion Ultrasound Bill," March 28, 2009.

17. Neela Banerjee, "Church Groups Turn to Sonogram to Turn Women From Abortions," *New York Times*, February 2, 2005.

18. Harrison, interview.

19. Sabin Russell, "First Fetal Surgery Survivor Finally Meets His Doctor," *San Francisco Chronicle*, May 5, 2005.

20. Michael Harrison, "Personal Perspective," *Fetal Diagnosis and Therapy*.

21. Casper, interview.

22. Pedro del Nido in interview with the author's team.

CHAPTER SEVEN: WHAT IS A MIRACLE?

1. Unless otherwise noted, information on Matthew Pfenninger's case comes from interviews with Jack Pfenninger and Matthew Pfenninger, conducted by the author and/or his team.

2. There are numerous studies to this effect. Not only do Americans pray a great deal, according to a 2004 National Institutes of Health Survey of more than 31,000 people, prayer is the most commonly used "alternative medicine." (*NIH newsletter*, http://nccam.nih.gov/news/newsletter/2005_winter/prayer.htm)

3. Herbert Benson and others, "Study of the therapeutic effects of intercessory prayer...," *American Heart Journal* 51, no. 4 (April 2006): 934–942.

4. Adam C. Randolph, Erin M. Tharalson, and Nooman Gilani, "Spontaneous regression of heptocellular carcinoma is possible and might have implications for future therapies," *European Journal of Gastroenterology & Hepatology* 20, no. 8 (August 2008): 804–809; Nooman Gilani in interview with the author's team.

5. Gilani, interview.

6. Jeanne Lenzer, "The Body Can Beat Terminal Cancer—Sometimes," *Discover*, August 21, 2007

7. Alcides Moreno's brother Edgar died in the same incident.

8. David Gorski in interview with the author's team.

9. Not uncommon for a blog, Respectful Insolence has changed its archiving process a number of times and it would not be surprising if it changed again. Rather than post a full link, anyone interested in reading the posts on medical miracles and Abraham Cherrix is encouraged to go to the main page, http://scienceblogs.com/insolence/ and run a search for the topic of their choice.

10. Wikipedia, http://en.wikipedia.org/wiki/Hoxsey_Therapy

11. Michael Hardy, "Kaine Signs Bills, Including 'Abraham's Law,'" *Richmond Times-Dispatch*, March 22, 2007

12. www.powerball.com

13. Unless otherwise noted, information on David Bailey's case comes from the following: interviews with David Bailey and Dr. Henry Friedman conducted by the author and/or his team, and correspondence with David Bailey.

14. Darrell Bigner in interview with the author; Dietmar Krex, "Long-term survival with glioblastoma multiforme," *Brain* 130, no. 10 (2007): 2596–2606.

15. Henry Friedman, interview.

16. Krex, "Long-term survival..." *Brain*, 130.

17. Henry Friedman, interview.

18. The most dramatic evidence of extended survival comes from

trials involving a vaccine that targets a substance EGFRvIII, produced by the tumor cells. It's discussed in more depth, a bit later in this chapter.

19. National Cancer Institute, http://www.cancer.gov/cancertopics/treatment/brain/malignantglioma

20. Roger Stupp, "Radiotherapy plus concomitant and adjuvant temozolomide for glioblastoma," *New England Journal of Medicine* 352, no. 10 (2005): 987–996.

21. Henry Friedman, interview.

22. John Sampson in interview with the author.

23. *Journal of Clinical Oncology*, 2008 ASCO Annual Meeting Proceedings (Post-Meeting Edition). Volume 26, Number 15S (May 20 Supplement). Abstract #2011.

24. Henry Friedman, interview.

25. Much of Bailey's music is available to hear at www.davidm-bailey.com

CHAPTER EIGHT: ANOTHER DAY

1. The account of Zeyad Barazanji's treatment is based on interviews with Barazanji and Dr. Stephan Mayer, and a reading of Barazanji's medical records.

2. Mayer, interview.

3. Wade Davis, *The Serpent and the Rainbow* (New York: Harper-Collins, 1986).

4. http://en.wikipedia.org/wiki/Wade_Davis

5. David Abel, "Line Between Life and Death Can Be Thin," *Boston Globe*, January 26, 2001.

6. A more detailed explanation of the bureaucratic catch-22 is laid out in Chapter One of this book.

7. Theresa Olasveengen and others, "Abstract 13: A prospective randomized controlled trial on the effects of intravenous drug administration on survival to hospital discharge

after out-of-hospital cardiac arrest," *Circulation*, 2008; 118:S_1447.

8. The program, *Brennpunkt*, is aired by the Norwegian broadcaster NRK. The story on the cardiac arrest experiment was reported on January 8, 2008.

9. Gilbert, interview.

10. Hans Husum and others, "Rural prehospital trauma systems improve trauma outcome in low-income countries; a prospective study from North Iraq and Cambodia," *Journal of Trauma* 54, no. 6 (2003): 1188–1196.

11. Robert Kastenbaum, *Death, Society, and Human Experience*, 7th edition (Boston: Allyn & Bacon, 2001).

Acknowledgments

AS A DOCTOR, reporter, husband, and father, I know it is the families of my patients that are often forgotten and overlooked. Over the last two years, we directly entered the lives of the characters in this book. We took valuable time, and asked for them to recount sometimes painful stories. We called on weekends, at night, and during holidays just to get another fact nailed down and to get the story straight. The children, parents, spouses, and other relatives were universally patient with us, and for that I thank you. I hope you think this book honors your loved one, and all those who cheat death.

I would also like to thank my colleague and good friend, Caleb Hellerman. This book would not have been possible without him and his passion. Not only is he a terrific and thoughtful writer, but he is as diligent a researcher as one can find. Caleb is also serving as the executive producer of *Cheating Death*, the documentary.

About the Author

SANJAY GUPTA, MD, is a practicing neurosurgeon and associate chief of neurosurgery at Grady Memorial Hospital and assistant professor at Emory University Hospital in Atlanta. He is a columnist for *Time* magazine and chief medical correspondent at CNN, where he plays an integral role in the network's medical coverage, including daily reports, the show *House Call with Dr. Sanjay Gupta,* and coverage of breaking medical news. He is featured in a weekly podcast on health issues called "Paging Dr. Gupta" and writes health news stories for CNN.com and CNNHealth.com. He is also a contributor to *60 Minutes* and the *Evening News with Katie Couric* on CBS.

Before joining CNN, Gupta was a neurosurgeon at the University of Tennessee's Semmes-Murphy clinic, and before that, at the University of Michigan Medical Center. He became partner of the Great Lakes Brain and Spine Institute in 2000 and in 1997 he was chosen as a White House Fellow, one of only fifteen fellows appointed. He served as special adviser to former first lady Hillary Rodham Clinton.

Gupta has been published in a variety of scientific journals and has received numerous accolades. He received the health communication achievement award from the American Medical Association in 2009 and his health reports swept all three health and medical awards in 2006—the first year the National Headliner Awards honored such journalism in a dedicated category. Also in 2006, he earned his first Emmy®, a Peabody, and the DuPont award.

In 2004, the Atlanta Press Club named Gupta "Journalist of the Year." He has won the Humanitarian Award from the National Press Photographers Association, a GOLD Award from the National Health Care Communicators, and the International Health and Medical Media award known as the "Freddie." His first book, *Chasing Life*, became a *New York Times* best seller and was also the subject of a one-hour documentary of the same name on CNN.

A board-certified neurosurgeon, Gupta is a member of several organizations, including the American Association of Neurological Surgeons, Congress of Neurological Surgeons, and the Council of Foreign Relations. He serves as a diplomat of the American Board of Neurosurgery as a Fellow in the American College of Surgery and is a certified medical investigator. Gupta is also a board member of the Lance Armstrong LiveStrong Foundation.